Authenticity is a valuable currency right now, and for every 'Cloud 9' photo spread or impossibly perfect first 'mother and baby' picture on Instagram, there is a new mother in the public eye who is not scared to tell it like it is. Hearing that celebrities have challenges adapting to postpartum life can help us muggles feel much more normal.

Here is a selection of some of my favourite postpartum quotes:

'I'm limping around. I'm still trying to figure out what [pregnancy] has done to my body, how it's changed it. What's temporary and what's permanent.' Hayden Panettiere, actor

'Is it alright if I admit that, after giving birth myself, I really didn't give a stuff that my belly felt like blancmange, and the last thing that I cared about was feeling beautiful? In fact, I found a sweet freedom in not caring. Shappi Khorsandi, comedian

'My body has more curves now, more folds, more softness, and all of that is the evidence of my biological powers.' Jodie Turner-Smith, actor

'I guess we anticipate or expect that our bodies will suddenly be back to what they were – but it really takes time. Often the conversation around the postpartum body is just around weight – but it's actually much more complicated than that. I've struggled with incontinence and prolapse and all the other glamorous parts of childbirth that no one really talks about – it's hard to feel confident when you're not sure your body will let you down.' Ashley James, DJ, influencer and TV personality

'It's amazing, two sneezes, I'm fine. Three, it's game over.' Kate Winslet, Oscar-winning actor, on incontinence

'I was back running about 12 days after giving birth to Isla, which was too soon. I was really excited and probably built the miles up too quickly, which is how I ended up with a stress fracture in my sacrum. I hadn't recovered from the trauma of the birth. I ended up not being able to run for three months afterwards, although 10 months after giving birth I did win the New York Marathon.' Paula Radcliffe, world champion runner

*'I can confirm postpartum life is 90% better when you don't rip to your butthole.'* Chrissy Teigen, American television personality, on her second postpartum experience

*'I don't think it was till he was probably like a year old and I was looking at my body and thinking why hasn't it gone back now? You know how people have their babies and then, like, a week later they'd just look back to normal? I didn't. I really didn't.'* Stacey Solomon, TV personality and national treasure (IMHO)

*'You're an entirely different person. But that transition to being an entirely different person isn't easy. That idea that any of that should be easy, and that should be seamless, I find it really offensive.'* Keira Knightley, actor*

*'For three months, I was walking around my house with a top knot, giant diaper, nipples bleeding. Like a defeated sumo wrestler.'* Ali Wong, comedian

*'It's not about "getting back" to where I was. It's about going forward to where I want to be. My postpartum journey will never end – I'll always have a prolapse to consider. But I feel the hard work is paying off (with a bit of help from 'Poppy' my pessary). I'm no longer scared about a bouncy castle, star jumps or racing my kids downhill. I feel I can live my life as I want to again.'* Sophie Power, sportsperson

*'I'm proud of my tummy. It pokes out a lot more than it used to, but I'm still coming back from having a baby. I just feel like this whole story about having a baby and coming back two days after and looking better than before is not teaching the right way or the natural way or the believable way.'* Serena Williams, tennis champion

*'It's the site of a miracle now.'* Kerry Washington

---

* Look up 'Kiera Knightley postpartum' for some other absolutely bang on truth-bombs about postpartum life and motherhood in general.

# YOUR POSTNATAL BODY

## A TOP-TO-TOE GUIDE TO CARING FOR YOURSELF AFTER PREGNANCY AND BIRTH

LYANNE NICHOLL

**None of the information included in this book is meant to replace advice, guidance and appointments with your healthcare team.**

# CONTENTS

# AUTHOR'S NOTE

I have never been happier in my body, and I have never been more content than I am now. I am saying this from the outset as, in this book, I am highlighting a range of challenging issues that I, and many other mothers, may have had to overcome. I may moan a fair bit. And I'm not going to apologise for that. Just because I feel blessed and filled with joy to have my boys, does not mean that I have to keep shtum about the physical rigours that pregnancy, birth and the postnatal period present. Equally, some mums don't feel content and filled with joy – at least some of the time – and may actually resent changes that have happened to their body. And, you know what, that's okay too. It is not anybody's job to police how we feel about our bodies at any point in our lives and becoming a mother does not change this. So – you do you! My hope is that this book will give you the tools to navigate your new postnatal body and empower you to create a plan for your optimal health. Beyond that, I also hope it will be a starting point for feeling acceptance of your body now you are a mother.

I talk about vaginas a fair bit in this book because, well, this is a postpartum book and vaginas are pretty central. I absolutely agree that we should know the correct anatomical names for our bodies, especially if we are talking to health professionals (to avoid confusion). However, I don't hold much truck with the idea that we cannot use euphemisms and nicknames for vaginas when we want to. People will say that we don't use 'silly' words for other parts of our bodies, but we do. Bonce, noggin, barnet fair, boobs, belly, funny bone – I could go on. I feel this book would be a bit dry if I was to be po-faced all the way through. And one thing you don't want a vagina to be is… dry.

## Post-Partum

*they told me i was pregnant*
*then told me i was glowing*
*then told me i was blooming*
*belly slowing growing life*
*i gave birth to a baby*
*i took the baby home*
*they told me she was beautiful*
*they told me, i agreed*
*my body wrapped in silence now*
*to lie and weep and bleed*

Hollie McNish

# INTRODUCTION

You matter. Your body matters. I am glad you picked up this book as this is the first step to regaining confidence in your body – and I absolutely don't mean that in a 'get fit quick' way. I mean it in the sense that you regain trust in your body and feel the best you possibly can about yourself.

While pregnant, you receive a glut of information on pregnancy symptoms – *what to expect when you're expecting*, if you will. But what about afterwards? What are the symptoms of 'postpartum'? Which are normal, which are worrying? This book aims to explain what is happening to your body now that your little bundle(s) have arrived, and how you can help yourself recover and thrive.

Ever since I had my first son in 2015, I have been flabbergasted by the lack of care and attention given to women's postnatal bodies. Aside from the unhealthy fixation on getting back in to 'pre-pregnancy' jeans, no one seems to give a rat's arse about what you have just been through. Pregnancy and birth may be everyday occurrences, but they are not easy, and the after-effects can be wide-ranging and sometimes difficult to live with. To (mis)quote Kiera Knightley, 'Birth happens every day. What's the big deal? So does death, but you don't have to pretend that's easy.' Women are often well prepared for pregnancy and the side-effects and symptoms that come with it, but can be blind-sided by a host of new symptoms that appear postnatally. This can be particularly hard after a difficult birth, if you don't have much support, or if you are struggling mentally and emotionally.

I still remember the postnatal period with my first son very clearly, despite surviving on about three hours' sleep a night – or maybe because of that. It was not easy. I was sore, leaky and overwhelmed and it was left solely up to me to research what was normal and what wasn't and create my own care pathway. That experience led me to start the Postnatal Health Community on social media and begin campaigning for better postnatal care. There are signs that things are improving (or there were pre-pandemic!) but we are still a long way from satisfactory care for women, and birthing people, after birth.

I hope to be able to empower you by increasing your knowledge about what the hell just happened and how to *really* look after yourself. You may feel that all of your attention needs to be on your baby or babies, and this notion may be perpetuated by friends, family, and even health professionals, but I am here to say: you matter. Taking care of your physical and mental health is paramount, not only because a healthy, happy mum is more likely to be able to cope with the demands of parenthood and enable her children to thrive, but because you are still the whole human being you were before, and you deserve to recover properly.

We should not take the current 'put up and shut up' culture sitting down – especially if you are currently sat on one of those inflatable doughnut rings. For too long there has been a casual disregard of women's bodies after birth, as if we have served our purpose as a vessel and are no longer of much value. There is a pervasive culture of 'well, this is just what happens after childbirth', particularly when it comes to things like urinary incontinence. Weeing your pants when you laugh, sneeze or run postpartum may be common, but it is not normal, and we have been sold a lie that it is. And the word 'sell' here is particularly pertinent. The adult continence industry is booming, faster than children's nappies. Well, 'oops moments' (sigh) are not part and parcel of becoming a mother. It's not our fault that we just put up with this – we haven't been told any different. There has been a wall of silence about the reality of postpartum bodies. The mothers who went before us just 'got on with it' because women are stoic, resilient and, unfortunately, accustomed to their health issues being minimised. But that changes now. With proper care postnatally, we can strengthen and support our bodies to recover – and maintain optimal physical health for life.

This book does not seek to diminish the importance of mental health postpartum. The statistics show how worryingly prevalent mental health issues are for new mothers. There are a significant number of books that address postnatal depression and anxiety. Far fewer deal with physical recovery post-birth. I am very firmly of the opinion that the two are interlinked in any case. The mind-body connection has long been proven and, from a personal perspective, I know my mood would have been significantly better had someone taken proper care of my physical self after my birth experience. As it was, my world had been turned upside down by the arrival of this heart-wrenchingly cute and vulnerable little baby. I was exhausted, battered and swollen but very much expected to 'just get on with it' and accept unquestioningly any changes to my body, no matter how painful they might be. Many mothers ride a wave of emotions in those early days and months, as I did, but how much more reassuring would it be if there was a plan in place to piece you back together? At the moment, that service does not really exist within our over-stretched maternity services and so I hope this book will be your helping hand.

One thing I really feel the need to stress from the off is that after five pregnancies and two births (one vaginal, one caesarean) – I have never felt happier with my body. This book contains an overwhelming list of things that *might* happen to your body and, if you are currently pregnant or hoping to become so, you'd be forgiven for thinking 'fuck that'! BUT, and this is a big but, not only may many of these things *not* happen to your body, but it is also critical to remember that your body has done a wonderful thing and needs love and appreciation. Equally you need to know when to push for more help, where to go and how to help your body heal optimally. I hope I succeed in showing you how to do this.

I think my positive/neutral attitude toward my body is partly because I thought that it might look and feel a lot worse after all I'd been through, but also because I was armed with the right information to take care of myself and I believe I am reaping the rewards of that. I don't look perfect (whatever that is), but the way I feel about my body is way more important than that 'perfect 10' image, and I feel pretty good about my 40-odd-year-old mum-bod – jiggly bits and all.

## A QUICK TOP-TO-TOE

Here is a brief rundown of the side-effects you *could* experience directly after birth or in the weeks, months and even years afterwards. I say 'could' because not all women experience the same side-effects. Some of you will be lucky and experience just a few, and hopefully not too drastically (I do look at those pictures of the Duchess of Cambridge on the steps of the Lindo Wing and think 'you poor woman' as *no one* escapes *all* the glorious after-effects!). Some of you will experience many of them, but do not panic – there are ways and means of dealing with them all. The important thing is to recognise what is normal and what is not.

| | |
|---|---|
| **Hair** | *postpartum hair loss, changes to hair* |
| **Head** | *postpartum headaches and migraines, jaw pain, dizziness* |
| **Brain** | *neurological changes* |
| **Hormones** | *mood changes, fatigue, night sweats* |
| **Eyes** | *changes to eyesight, dry eyes, floaters* |
| **Nose** | *changes to sense of smell, rhinitis, size* |
| **Mouth** | *changes to your teeth and gums, oral thrush from antibiotics, taste changes* |
| **Spine (neck, back)** | *pain, postural issues, recovering from spinal block/epidural* |
| **Heart** | *hypertension (high blood pressure), low blood pressure* |
| **Blood** | *lochia, how you feel after blood loss and/or blood transfusion, taking blood thinners* |
| **Breasts** | *swollen, sore breasts, leaking, mastitis, cracked nipples, nipple thrush, changing shape and size* |
| **Ribs** | *expanded ribcage* |
| **Stomach and core** | *how your belly feels after birth (including phantom kicks), diastasis recti, gut reaction to taking antibiotics, general weakness, stretch marks* |
| **Hips and pelvis** | *pain, postural issues, prolapse, pubic bone injuries, pelvic floor issues (including incontinence)* |
| **Uterus** | *cramps, infection, shrinking back, endometriosis after c-section, painful or heavy periods* |
| **Vagina** | *tears, haematoma, episiotomies, pain, dyspareunia, infection* |
| **Bum** | *constipation, coccydynia, haemorrhoids, fissures, wind, incontinence, prolapse, pain* |
| **Legs** | *varicose veins, spider veins, deep vein thrombosis* |
| **Feet** | *swelling, fallen arches, bigger feet* |

# CHAPTER 1

# RECOVERY AFTER BIRTH – THE FIRST 24 HOURS

The first 24 hours after birth can be a bit of a blur. Your birth experience can, obviously, profoundly affect how you feel in the first few days and beyond. Whether you had a long labour, trauma, blood loss, or a planned caesarean section/abdominal birth – suffice to say birthing a baby and the subsequent recovery is not a walk in the park.

Firstly, I hope it went well! If there were any complications at all, with you and/or with your baby, I recommend a thorough debrief with the obstetrics and midwifery teams before you are discharged. Your health is your wealth, please don't be fobbed off.

So what might you experience in those first 24 hours? Well, you'll likely experience some pain, mostly around your vagina or your stomach – depending on what the mode of birth was. You may also experience nipple pain if you are beginning to breastfeed. You can request pain relief! I don't remember having much after my first (vaginal) birth, even though I was very sore, but I did alternate paracetamol and oramorph (a kind of morphine that is only available in hospitals) after my caesarean birth.

My own experience, both times, was that I felt like I had been hit by a train after giving birth. I know it is not the case for everyone. I have heard of women who feel euphoric after birth, but I felt exhausted, achy and swollen. If you lose a lot of blood, you may feel particularly tired. If you needed an epidural or spinal block, whether as part of a vaginal birth or abdominal birth, you will need to regain the feeling in your legs before you can get up and move about. You may be wearing surgical stockings to help prevent blood clots. These are neither snazzy nor comfortable. If you have had any kind of surgery, you may struggle to walk in those first 24 hours – rest assured, this is normal.

It will feel very debilitating and frustrating not being able to walk, particularly if you don't have a birth partner with you. If this is the case, please flag it to your midwifery team as you will need help both tending to yourself (such as going the loo/showering) and your baby. Trapped wind is a common complaint in those early hours, so your stomach might feel swollen and sore, and remember the pain from trapped wind can manifest in odd areas of your body, such as your shoulder! You will bleed from your vagina after any type of birth and this blood and discharge is called lochia.

Red flags, which you should raise with your healthcare provider, include excessive blood loss, fever (chills), hives, oozing from incision sites, foul-smelling discharge, cloudy urine which is difficult to pass, severe pain, shortness of breath, feeling disorientated or a sense of doom, severe headaches and/or dizziness, and a throbbing or red/hot calf (this can indicate a deep vein thrombosis, which is a blood clot).

Don't let the above alarm you. Some women will feel good and 'well' after birth.

## POSTNATAL SYMPTOMS – OR BLOOD, SWEAT AND TEARS

Below is a pretty long list, though not exhaustive, of symptoms we may experience in the initial postpartum period. Should we call them 'symptoms' if we are not 'sick'? Well, despite pregnancy being a natural state and not an illness, it often does create 'symptoms' (nausea, anyone?) in your body. Likewise, even if you do not have any conditions to contend with, the immediate postnatal period will result in some symptoms in your body.

### Hormonal changes

The hormonal Molotov cocktail that happens straight after birth is perhaps the biggest hormonal shift to happen in a short period of time that any human will ever experience. How do you like them apples? This is a big deal. Both your progesterone (the 'pregnancy' hormone which helps establish and nourish an embryo) and oestrogen (a hormone which aids with womb lining and developing organs in the foetus), which have been so critical in helping you build your baby, plummet and very soon are back to baseline pre-pregnancy levels.

At the same time, your body should be flooded with oxytocin (the 'bonding' hormone) and prolactin (originally named because of its function in enabling lactation). The way I am envisaging this is as a rollercoaster. During labour/pre-surgery you're at the very top and then once you deliver your baby you go plunging downwards at breakneck speed – only to swoop back up for the next loop. No wonder you don't know which way is up for that first couple of weeks. These dramatic hormonal changes, as well as emotional and environmental factors, can make you feel tired and weepy and can increase feelings of anxiety. Hormonal shifts can also affect your skin, joints and bones. Oxytocin should help you feel 'loved up' and able to bond with your baby. Oxytocin and prolactin can, however, be affected by trauma and blood loss. This is why women having caesareans are often told (or were in the past) that their hormone levels after surgery may adversely affect bonding and breastfeeding. To balance this view, I lost more blood with my vaginal birth than I did with my (planned) caesarean, and I found breastfeeding and the availability of milk easier after my caesarean. As with most things, it is multi-factorial and there are many things – both environmental and physiological – which can affect the production of milk and your mood.

Oxytocin levels are at their highest level for one hour after the birth, which is one reason why it is called 'the golden hour'. Your elevated oxytocin helps the uterus contract, which expels the placenta and cuts off the blood supply to it, helping to prevent a postpartum haemorrhage. It also enables the release of milk (colostrum initially) from your nipple; the infant's suckling action boots the oxytocin into action to 'eject milk'. Clever stuff. You can 'up' your oxytocin release with eye contact and comfortable stroking of the skin. This wonderful hormone also acts as an anti-inflammatory, increases your pain threshold, induces calm, and will warm up the skin on your chest for your newborn to snuggle in to. Oxytocin will likely remain raised, although gradually decrease, for about eight weeks postpartum. Studies have not yet concluded whether oxytocin remains higher or lower in lactating mothers,[1] but there is a theory that oxytocin release by way of breastfeeding may paint part of the picture as to why breastfeeding mothers experience lower incidence of diabetes and cardiovascular issues.

### Lochia

Lochia is pronounced lock-ee-ya. Yes, more blood for us women to contend with. But we're used to it by now, right? Lochia is the discharge that comes out of your vagina after you have given birth. It is a mixture of blood, mucous and uterine tissue. Every woman that gives birth will experience this whether it was a c-section or vaginal birth. The amounts of blood and colour, consistency and so on will vary – as will the amount of time you bleed for – but, on average, it lasts for two to six weeks postpartum. With my first child I had heavy lochia for six weeks and with my second I had a very small amount for four weeks. You may notice heavier bleeding if you are breastfeeding as the uterus contracts as you feed. This bleeding should not be painful or smelly, you should not develop a temperature with it and very large clots should be flagged to your healthcare provider. A significant bleed, which soaks through more than one pad, and has much larger clots, should be investigated as there is a small chance it could be postpartum haemorrhage and not just lochia. Too much physical exertion can also increase lochia, so be mindful of that.

### Postpartum haemorrhage

A postpartum haemorrhage means you lose a pint, or more, of blood after the birth, but it is not very common (statistics vary but it is less than 10% prevalence) and most will happen within 24 hours of birth. You should speak up if you feel you are losing too much blood as health practitioners can help prevent a bigger bleed. Losing too much blood could lead to anaemia and other complications. If you have had excessive blood loss (normally this means over two pints of blood) then you may have had manual help to stop the bleeding, either in theatre or in the birth room, or you may have been given a blood transfusion. How your body reacts to blood loss is relative to each individual. Midwife Sophie Hiscock (The Village Midwife) told me that some women deal well with significant blood loss, whereas a smaller amount of blood loss can more adversely affect someone else.

If you have had a transfusion, then you should have been given a leaflet which lists possible (rare) reactions that can occur up to about two weeks after the transfusion. It is important that you (and your partner, if you have one) take note of these possible side-effects as some can be serious and you would need hospital care. You are likely to feel very fatigued if you have experienced significant blood loss. There is also such a thing as a secondary postpartum haemorrhage, which can occur after the initial 24 hours and up to 12 weeks after birth and will be most likely related to some of the placenta not having come away (retained placenta). Do keep an eye on your blood loss. If it is significant you may need to be tested for anaemia, which can be simply treated with iron supplements.

### Infections

Infections do happen but are not hugely common and can be treated easily with antibiotics. Between 10-15% of vaginal and abdominal births will result in infection. You will be monitored if you are in hospital. Do keep an eye on your temperature, any swelling or pain which seems excessive or unusual, weeping wound sites, red patches on your breasts, cystitis-type symptoms and also any foul-smelling discharge (including the lochia). Bacteria can also travel to your urinary tract, causing a urinary-tract infection (UTI), or to your uterus causing endometritis, which sounds like endometriosis but is something entirely different. Endometritis is inflammation of the womb, so be aware of unusual tenderness in your lower abdomen. Do flag signs of possible infection, as the quicker it is seen to the quicker and easier the recovery will be.

### Pain

I've asked you to look out for tenderness above. Knowing what a normal level of pain and discomfort is after giving birth is definitely a bit of a minefield – so, although the below are common, do raise it with your healthcare provider if something doesn't feel right or feels excessively painful. You might have pain in all sorts of areas after birth, but the most common ones would be pain from a wound (perineal tear, episiotomy or c-section), contracting uterus pains, swollen breasts, and nipple pain from breastfeeding.

- **Pain from a tear or episiotomy** (surgical cut to the perineum) can vary from person to person. Some women only have minor pains for a short period of time and others will have pain or discomfort at this site for weeks, months or years. Pain for weeks is in the range of normal, but pain for months and years, however, is not and should be flagged to your healthcare provider. Any oozing, or strange smell would need to be investigated. I had quite a bad tear after my first son and found sitting normally really uncomfortable for about two weeks as I was so swollen.

- **Pain from a c-section scar** will, again, vary with each individual but there will likely be at least a few days of significant pain. Most women I have spoken to who have had c-sections say they notice considerable improvement after two weeks. For me, it was three. I was hobbling around the bed for a good week, and I took every pain med going.

- **Uterus cramping.** Well, NO ONE told me that I'd get period-style cramps AFTER the birth. Your uterus has expanded by up to 500 times its normal size in pregnancy (wowee!) and needs to contract back down to its usual size. If you breastfeed, this might happen quicker and with stronger contractions that feel like labour or menstrual pains, as suckling on the breast releases a hormone which helps the uterus to contract. If this is your second baby or you've had a particularly large baby, the uterus may be slightly more stretched which can make cramps feel a bit more intense. They may also be more painful if you've had a caesarean. Luckily, mine weren't too bad but some women find them toe-curling. Either way, they shouldn't last long. This 'involution' (shrinking back and returning to normal size) of the uterus, and also the cervix and vagina, takes approximately six weeks and is also what helps pump out the lochia.

- **Breast and nipple pain.** Your boobs are about to get huge. This was a big thing for me. After years of feeling slightly forlorn about my tangerines, I was about to get melons. It was both very exciting and excruciatingly painful. They felt hard and very tender. This normally happens on day three, when your milk comes in, although it can be delayed by things like trauma, excessive blood loss and/ or surgery. Large, tender breasts are normal. Hot breasts with red or discoloured patches and with you running a temperature are not, however, as these are signs of mastitis (more on this later). Engorgement can make your breasts and nipples feel particularly hard and uncomfortable. Nipple pain will very likely go hand in hand with establishing breastfeeding. I could write an entire book on breastfeeding and the myriad of issues we experienced but suffice to say that I feel women are currently being done a huge disservice in being encouraged to breastfeed but without enough support or signposting – or, indeed, honesty about its challenges. I am glad I was able to breastfeed my sons, but it was a long and tricky road with both and it started with some gnarled up nipples. Despite what you might read via Dr Google, the issues are *unlikely* to be nipple thrush and *very likely* to be related to the latch (however good it looks from the outside). If it *is* thrush it will likely be characterised by stabbing pains at the front of the breast, itching, shiny or flaky nipples and burning nipple pain. It is more likely to occur if you have thrush elsewhere in the body (common after antibiotic use) or if the baby has thrush. Pain from a bad latch or if the baby has tongue-tie is more likely to cause bleeding and pinched or 'wedge-shaped' nipples. Blanched (white) nipples after a feed can also be caused by a bad latch which might be caused by a vasospasm and/or 'mammary constriction syndrome'. These things happen when blood flow to the breast and nipple becomes restricted. You may have also heard of the phrase 'let down': this is not only an Australian sitcom, which takes a witty and honest look at motherhood, but something that happens as your milk prepares to leave your breast. As your baby suckles, the nerves in your breast are stimulated, sending signals to your milk ducts to release milk. Most women experience this as a tingling sensation, but it can be painful for some. Others don't feel it at all. It is important to note that while breastfeeding, if you choose to do it and are able to, might start off being uncomfortable, it should not be painful – especially after the first couple of weeks. If you are keen to continue to breastfeed but are experiencing pain in your breasts or nipples, please do contact your healthcare provider and/or use some of the resources at the back of this book.

- **Back pain.** This can be as a result of a spinal block/epidural or from exertion, exhaustion, awkward birthing position, or a back-to-back labour, for example. Muscle spasms after regional anaesthesia can last for days, or even weeks.

The above are the most common sites for pain. However, below are potential red flags, so take note if you have pain in *your calf* – this can be indicative of a deep vein thrombosis (blood clot) and these can be dangerous. Seek emergency medical advice if your calf is tight, hot, red, swollen and/or painful, *especially* if accompanied by shortness of breath. Also if you have pain in *your chest* – gasping for breath, unusual coughing and chest pain can be indicative of a pulmonary embolism (blood clot on the lung) or a symptom of preeclampsia (although giving birth usually resolves preeclampsia, this is not always the case) and both of these should be investigated immediately.

Any extreme pain should be flagged to a health professional.

To think for aeons we've been called the 'weaker sex'. Dude, please! Anyway, that's a whole other legion of books.

### Tummy

I have been heartened in recent years to see more and more women posting realistic pictures of the days and weeks after birth which show a distended tummy. It takes time for your uterus to shrink, and some people will still look pregnant for quite a while after the birth. Your skin and tissues have all stretched and you can end up with quite a floppy/jiggly/squishy tummy at first. Most women experience a degree of 'diastasis recti', which is when your abdominal muscles separate to allow room for the growing baby. You may feel weak in your core for quite some time after the birth, particularly if you had a c-section, as the incision will have involved your stomach muscles being moved about. Some women may find the 'empty' or deflated feeling of their jiggly belly quite disconcerting.

### Sweat

Just under a third of women will experience 'hot flushes' in the postpartum period.[2] Your hormones are instructing your body to get rid of excess fluid that you were carrying during pregnancy. If you had intravenous fluids (IV fluids, also called 'a drip') during labour/birth then you will also have this excess water to lose. This is why you may sweat (and also wee) more. Hot flushes can often take the form of night sweats and you may wake with soaked sheets, which can be uncomfortable. Many women find they are just generally a bit sweatier and pongier after birth. I took breastfeeding supplements that included fenugreek which made my sweat smell really strange. There is a hypothesis that your sweat may smell a little bit more as newborns' sight and hearing is not fully developed and they navigate their way to your breast via odour. Your areola secretes oils and milk, which will attract the newborn to suckle, but perhaps your new underarm whiff is also a little signpost on where best to head for a drink. It's temporary, so don't sweat it. All of this should settle down within two to six weeks.

### Headaches

Approximately 40% of all women report postpartum headaches[3] - so, yay! Not only is your foof/tummy all ouchy and you're likely exhausted, but now you have a pounding head! Well, this is one thing I did not have, so let's hope you're in that 60% with me. These headaches can often be attributed to dehydration, tiredness, tension, hormone shifts – the usual culprits. Occasionally, there will be something more to them that could signal a reaction to medication or a symptom of preeclampsia, which can occur even after giving birth.[4] A headache caused by preeclampsia can often be felt right across the head, it may pulse and worsen with activity and may be accompanied by blurred or altered vision. Preeclampsia is a medical emergency, so get checked out if you experience any of the above.

Sometimes regional anaesthesia can cause your headache. A *postdural puncture headache* is a specific kind of severe headache which can occur after an epidural or spinal block. Your brain and spinal cord are contained in a bag of fluid. The bag is called the dura and the fluid is called the cerebro-spinal fluid. If the dura is punctured, some of this fluid may leak out which can cause pressure changes to the brain, which in turn causes the headaches. It feels worse if you're upright and only gets better when lying down flat. You may also experience neck pain, sickness and/or an aversion to bright lights. Some patients will liken it to a migraine. It could start between one day and one week after the spinal or epidural injection.[5] If you experience a severe headache in the days or weeks after childbirth, it should be flagged to your healthcare provider urgently. If you experience dizziness or nausea at the same time, it might be a medical emergency and so you should treat it as such.

### Haemorrhoids

Oh, the glamour! Yes, piles really are a pain in the bum! I remember asking a good friend for her honest advice as she gave birth weeks before I was due. 'You may get piles from pushing' she said – as well as some other choice phrases and expletives. Many, if not most, women already have 'piles' from carrying a baby through pregnancy due to the additional weight, but labour and birth can, indeed, exacerbate them. A haemorrhoid is a painful swelling of a vein, or veins, in your rectum (back passage). They can be caused by the pressure of extra weight, increased blood volume, constipation (or other pushing!) and those fabulous – but mischievous – hormones! Haemorrhoids can cause pain, rectal itching, bleeding after having a bowel movement, or a swollen area around the anus. Some, luckily, will give you no bother, and will likely reduce in size and annoyance in the weeks after the birth.

### Fissures

I hate to be the bearer of bad news, but there's more. Haemorrhoids' fun bed-fellows are 'fissures'. Fissures are skin tears in the anus or the anal canal. These are about as fun as they sound. As with piles, fissures can be caused by childbirth or constipation and, sometimes, by diarrhoea. Those with Irritable Bowel Syndrome (IBS) may be more susceptible. Fissures can be very painful, and it is best to 'keep regular' to avoid making them worse. Sitz baths (a warm, shallow bath, often with salt added) and painkillers may help in the short term, but if they're really bothering you, then contact your GP as they will be able to prescribe treatment to alleviate symptoms.

### Bladder and bowel

There is a reason why midwives make sure you pee and poo before they discharge you. Both urinating and emptying your bowels can be more difficult in the immediate postpartum period. This can be for a number of reasons: swelling, nerve damage, muscles that have been stretched, urinary retention, constipation and/or the effects of anaesthesia or pain relief. Your bowels might be particularly sluggish if you've had a c-section (as abdominal surgery puts your bowel into 'quiet mode') and you may particularly struggle to pee if you've had a catheter inserted. Equally you may leak urine in the first few days after the birth and have difficulty controlling wind. It might also sting when you wee after a vaginal birth, and you might feel nervous about your first poo. All of this is normal. I will go into more detail later in the book about what is normal/not normal with regards to pelvic matters and bladder and bowel function, but for the first few days go easy on yourself, try to relax and understand that your body has just gone through a major upheaval and might be a bit shy with the peeing and pooping initially – but maybe not with trumping, annoyingly. Especially if you've had a caesarean. Windy City. Trapped wind is really common and it can manifest itself with pain in weird places like your ribs or shoulder. Your pelvic floor will likely have been stretched or compromised through the weight gain of pregnancy and the rigours of birth. If you're accustomed to doing pelvic floor exercises, you may find it harder to engage these muscles in the days and weeks after birth. Don't worry too much as, with time and practice, these should become much stronger again.

### Oedema

All the swelling you get in late pregnancy goes straight away, right? You deflate like a balloon? Ummm, not quite! It takes a little time. The progesterone increase in pregnancy will have caused some fluid retention already, then if you add on top of that increased blood flow from the exertions of labour or to incision sites and a build-up of IV fluids – you may feel a little bit like a water balloon again. Most of the swelling will occur in your hands and feet – although I distinctly remember having a very puffy face after my firstborn. Your body will rid you of this extra fluid via weeing and sweating more than usual. Excessive swelling that does not subside should be flagged to your healthcare team.

### Reactions to antibiotics

If you had any type of surgical intervention, or if you tested positive for Group Strep B, you will have been given antibiotics. Antibiotics can play havoc with your gut, so you may experience nausea, vomiting, diarrhoea or IBS-type symptoms. Sometimes taking antibiotics can result in thrush, so watch out for itchiness and pain in the vaginal area, nipples or mouth. Oral thrush can give you a black tongue. Like I had. Bringing sexy back, y'all.

### Tender areas due to injections

You may be a little tender in your back if you had a spinal block/epidural. Also, if you have been prescribed anticoagulants (blood thinners) after surgery, you may also begin to get sore patches from the injection sites. I needed to inject myself for over 20 weeks throughout pregnancy and beyond, so I know how tender it can get. Make sure you mix up the injection site (you can use wodges of fat on either thigh or either side of your stomach) so that you are not always injecting in the same site; try to grab as much fat as you can and do the injection quickly rather than slowly and all this should help a little.

This book is not exhaustive and if anything seems 'off' do contact your healthcare team (midwife, health visitor, GP or hospital, if you are still under their care).

## YOUR IMMEDIATE RECOVERY – HOW TO LOOK AFTER YOURSELF AND ACCESS THE BEST CARE FOR YOUR WHOLE SELF

OK, so there's all this blood, pain, sweat and tears. And this is *after* the birth. Give me some good news, woman! I get it, this might not be what you want to hear. And you might just be the kind of woman who springs out of bed the day after having a baby and does a pirouette. But many of us aren't. I wasn't. I believe forewarned is forearmed. There is a lot you can do to prepare for your healing and recovery: even just mentally being aware and tuned in to the fact that you may be out of action for a while can help.

Let's talk first about the stuff you can have in your hospital bag and at home. Like most new mothers, you will likely have thought more about what the new baby needs than you. You may have spent hundreds sprucing up a nursery and buying booties and teddies. But the fact is that your baby needs very little in the first few days and weeks. Ask a friend or do an internet search on what to pack for your baby. And now let's concentrate on you. You need quite a few things to help you not only feel comfortable, but also strong and ready for the mammoth undertaking that is motherhood. If ever there is a time to put yourself first, it is now. Putting some thought into what you might need will take the heat off when you are (likely) all consumed by your scrumptious new addition.

## HOSPITAL BAG FOR YOU:

- Maternity pads: very absorbent pads that you'll need to change regularly to avoid infection. Take more than you think you will need. If you're eco-conscious, you can buy pads made out of eco-friendly materials, or even use washable reusable pads. Tampons and menstrual cups should not be used for lochia.
- Mesh pants – some women prefer those big mesh pants that come with absorbent maternity pads attached. I think I recall the Unmumsy Mum, Sarah Turner, was a particular fan of these.
- Huge pants – the bigger and more Granny-ish the better – to hold the huge maternity pads in place. They also feel more comfortable on your abdomen, whether you've had a c-section or not.
- Trousers with elasticated waists – ditto the above.
- Breast pads: helpful for absorbing leaking milk and soothing sore nipples. Reusable ones might be more comfortable. I liked the silk-lined ones.
- Nipple shields/covers – I didn't use shields as they didn't feel comfortable for me, but many mothers swear by them. These are (usually) plastic teats you wear over your own nipples to help relieve pain when your baby is latched on. It's worth noting that if you use shields, you may need help from a breastfeeding supporter while you establish breastfeeding. It might also be worth looking into nipple covers or shells for between feeds, like ones made out of silver (which has healing properties). With any of these things, hygiene is really important to avoid infection (remember bugs love warm, dark, moist areas) and it is also important to ensure nipples get enough air between feeds initially.
- Pillow – taking my own pillow (plus one for my partner) was a game-changer for me. Hospital pillows are generally a bit crap. I took a huge feeding pillow, and it was very comfy.

- Eye mask and ear plugs – in the hope you might get some sleep, while your birth partner watches your baby.
- Water bottle – a sports one would really help both while in labour and if you have any pain or wound afterwards that will mean lying flat is best. Also helpful for squeezing water on to your bits as you wee.
- Chewing gum and peppermint tea – essential if you've had a c-section for getting rid of trapped wind. There are reports that drinking large quantities of peppermint tea can reduce breastmilk supply, but there is scant research to support this. However, it's easy to try cutting it out if you do encounter supply issues.
- Healthy snacks (nuts, oat bars, dried fruit) – to help keep energy levels up and also help with early bowel movements.
- A hang-up wash bag – so you don't need to bend your poor, knackered body in the shower.
- Flip-flops: a postpartum verruca on top of everything else is a right ball-of-the-foot-ache. Take it from one who knows!
- Stretchy bras and button down tops if planning to breastfeed.
- A shawl – or something similar if you're shy about breastfeeding afterwards. I wasn't but I also wasn't particularly happy about next door's Dad keeping coming in the wrong booth when I was nursing.
- Multivitamins – you probably have some prenatal supplements left over. You can use these.
- Probiotics – very helpful for avoiding things like oral thrush or a dodgy tummy if you've had antibiotics.
- Arnica pills. Whether you're 'into' homeopathy or not, these tablets have got a good reputation for helping to ease swelling.
- A clip-on fan. Hospitals can get very hot, and this can help keep you cool.
- A tennis ball – for rolling over aching muscles.
- A phone charger with an extra-long lead (if you know, you know).
- A Do Not Disturb sign – for if you're lucky enough to get a private room at a hospital, or for when you get home and are not quite ready for visitors (or postmen knocking during a nap!)

## RECOVERING AT HOME OR IN HOSPITAL

Your immediate recovery (the days and weeks after delivery) might take place in hospital, or at home, or a mixture of the two depending on where and how you gave birth. Women can be discharged from six hours after birth if it was uncomplicated and in a birth centre, but the average would probably be 24–48 hours. I honestly don't know how to feel about this. While being at home can definitely be more conducive to quiet and rest, in most cases it seems awfully early to be cast adrift from medical professionals – especially if you have had any complications. That said, recovery in hospital can be hampered by noise, lack of nutritious food and just being in unfamiliar surroundings. Some women who have homebirths do not need to go to hospital afterwards at all, but you, your midwife and your health visitor should keep an eye on your recovery even if all went well at the birth. I'd wager that in most circumstances, recovering at home is preferable and more effective, but we should not rush to discharge postpartum women. If you are not ready, or anything does not feel right, stay and ask to be examined or speak with a doctor. Despite being tired and overwhelmed, your instincts will still be sharp so try to pause and listen to your body. You are not being a nuisance. It is better to be discharged slightly later, in full health, than to be re-admitted.

If you need to have a longer stay in hospital, make sure you stay hydrated and well-nourished (so do stock up your hospital bag and ask visitors – if you want them at all – to bring nutritious snacks) and that your bed linen is kept fresh and clean. Again, you are not being a nuisance. I know it can feel like it when our maternity units are so understaffed and stretched but think of it like this – creating optimal healing and recovery for you could mean less reliance on the NHS in the future. So, do ask your midwives and health assistants for help with meals (if you have accidentally missed the trolley), changing sheets, speaking with a consultant, keeping clean, staying on top of pain relief and so on.

Before you are discharged, pause and ask yourself if you feel well and if you need advice on pain management or signposting to help for postnatal mental health, physical health (such as pelvic floor issues) or breastfeeding. When I asked an obstetrician-gynaecologist what she felt a woman should ask before being discharged from hospital, she noted that ideally women should be prepped in the antenatal period so there shouldn't be any need to ferret around in her newly mushed brain (my words, not hers!) for a checklist. I get the sentiment, but it is worth trying to take advantage of the one time you get easy (ish) access to a dedicated multi-disciplinary maternity care team as, currently in the UK, once you are discharged care becomes quite siloed and there can be frustrating waiting times.

Definitely adhere to the nurse/midwife's insistence that you urinate and open your bowels before you go home. You don't want to have to return to hospital because of retention/impaction issues. Two of the women I spoke with for this book became chronically constipated and needed to be readmitted, and one developed a serious urinary tract infection from urine retention, so don't let that happen if you can possibly help it. You may be nervous about your first poo, whatever your mode of birth. You may want to ask for lactulose, or a similar stool softener, to help you if you've had stitches anywhere. Drinks lots of water (or prune juice if necessary). Try to relax and breathe deeply on the toilet and do not strain, as this will make haemorrhoids worse. Midwife Sophie Hiscock recommends holding a clean maternity pad on your stitches when you wee or poo, just for extra reassurance (although the likelihood of you tearing any stitches by going to the toilet is infinitesimal – Sophie has never heard of it happening on her shifts). If it stings when you wee, then pouring warm water on your nether regions as you go will likely help. Some women can only pee in the shower initially, which you will be able to do at home. Midwives usually want to measure your urine output, to ensure it is at a healthy level, so don't be surprised if you're given a natty little cardboard box to stick under *your* box when you go. Equally, ensure any wounds are not infected (check smell and pain levels) and it is okay to get any stitches double-checked before you leave. My midwife also insisted on giving me a strong dose of painkillers for my car journey after my c-section, which I will be forever grateful for.

Once home, there are things you can do to make the first few days more comfortable. In other cultures, the postnatal period is a sacred time of rest, relaxation and nourishment – with other women and family members looking after the new mother. There is a concept, which was once prevalent and is now gaining more traction again, called 'confinement'. It is a period of time, which differs from culture to culture, in which the mother generally stays indoors, often in bed most of the time, and is fed warming foods and fluids. The word 'confinement' conjures up something of a prison scenario though, and, while the promotion of rest and being cared for is crucial, some women may find confinement, in its strictest sense, too stifling or isolating. However, I definitely think there are lessons to be taken from our ancestors and other cultures regarding this critical period of time. Our culture promotes a 'bouncing back to normal' ethos which simply isn't achievable, or even desirable, for most. We are not accustomed to honouring our bodies throughout our lives, and definitely not postpartum. But, if we did, it could pay dividends for our current and future health – and for the family unit as a whole.

I was told to get out of the house as soon as possible after the birth. I hated that first trip out. Everything felt too loud and bright, I was still sore, and my baby looked too small and vulnerable in his pram. I didn't like the physical distance between us, and my instincts were screaming at me to go home and cocoon, but I felt like I was being over-dramatic and wimpy. I should have listened to my gut as the trip out was uncomfortable and upsetting. A week or so later I was happily going for little walks in the fresh air with my baby in a sling, while that first trip had felt too much, too soon, and left me feeling like I was doing something wrong to have found something so 'every day' so difficult.

There are conflicting reports online as to whether 'confinement' can lessen instances of postpartum depression or trigger it. I think, should you decide to try it, that you need to set the boundaries yourself and not have them imposed on you. Some of the traditions are thousands of years old and simply not sustainable or applicable to our changed environment. In the Chinese confinement model a female relative will likely be on hand to help 'pamper' you through the first 40 days after birth. Although my friend, Jane, who is a first-generation Chinese-Brit, baulked at not being allowed ice-cream, as the traditional practice forbids cold foods. The long 'lying-in' stage is similar in Indian, other South Asian, and African traditions. Midwife Sundas Khalid told me that she feels that women who adhere to this tradition (and are looked after and even 'waited on' for 40 days) are erroneously thought of as 'princesses' here, while it is the norm in the South Asian community.

There are pockets of this type of practice in Europe. In Holland, all women have a state-funded *Kraamverzorgster* for two weeks, who comes to your home and performs medical checks on mother and baby, helps families adapt to the newest member and undertakes household chores and cooking. In the UK, we used to have a similar type of role, as outlined by Sophie Messager in her wonderful book *Why Postnatal Recovery Matters*, but now we don't get this type of state-funded help. We can, however, hire 'postpartum doulas' to fulfil a similar role. If this sounds like the preserve of the wealthy, it's worth knowing that Doula UK runs a scheme whereby those from lower income backgrounds can access help for free or for a reduced fee. The Motherhood Group, founded by social entrepreneur Sandra Igwe, is also on hand to help black mothers access postpartum (or birth) doulas and counsellors if they are experiencing financial hardship. Alternatively, if you felt comfortable doing so, you could ask for friends and family to contribute to some time with a postnatal doula instead of buying baby gifts.

I don't know about you, but I feel like so much about the modern world is out of step with what we need: mind, body and soul. And never was this more apparent to me than in my postpartum days. These days are built for lying low and bedding in as a family, but our hectic 'productivity-focused' lives these days make it seem like this is indulgent or in some way a failing. I hope this changes. I truly believe that if we invest in new mothers, and birthing people, at this critical juncture in their lives, we are setting up the strongest foundation for future health.

Sophie Hiscock, who still works bank shifts as a midwife in a busy London maternity ward, has recently set up an amazing enterprise whereby she establishes antenatal and postnatal support groups, which focus on getting mothers back to optimal health. She is 'The Village Midwife'. We had a great chat about this project, her general experience as a midwife (I'm in awe of what they achieve, with so little resource and support) and her own recovery. Sophie had a difficult birth and postpartum period, exacerbated by becoming a single mum before the birth of her son. From this adversity, she is creating a wonderful new structure of support for new mums, and I asked her to share her 'postnatal plan' with me (see below). We both lamented how long women spend on birth plans (to be clear, I am absolutely in favour of birth plans!) without a second thought as to how they will manage their postpartum healing and recovery. Once we begin to see planning for this period become mainstream, we might begin to see the culture shift we so desperately need. This is a time to honour your body, conserve your energy, form new bonds and rest, rest, rest.

## MEAL TRAIN

In 2019 a couple from Philadelphia posted a request on the US-based 'Meal Train' website, which listed all of the meals they would love to accept from neighbours once their first baby arrived. It went viral because the meal list was extensive, niche and probably quite expensive. People were outraged. It's quite funny what people do and do not get outraged by. The decimation of our planet and 1% of our population hoarding 50% of global wealth – pah! Piffle. But a scared new Dad asking for some granola? *How very dare he?* Jesting aside, it is actually a lovely concept, which doula Laura Rice alerted me to, but this particular guy perhaps went a little OTT for some. If your local community does not have anything like this, and many don't, then you could politely ask local friends and family how they'd feel about setting a meal train up for you. They could use a shared calendar to mark when they could drop off a meal for you and everyone would know when, and maybe what, to provide. I know some people will find this idea 'princessy' – but since when was providing food and sustenance for each other considered such a tall order? It could simply be 'extra' portions of something you are already cooking, rather than the Roasted Sweet Potato Wraps with caramelised onion and avocado that 'Meal Train Dad' requested – as delicious as they sound.

## MOVE HOME – A CONSIDERATION

Hear me out!

Three separate conversation strands led me to this suggestion. I was out for a meal with a new friend, Holly, and she told me how something that had helped her in the early days postpartum was going and staying at her mum's one night a week. The fresh sheets, having someone to hold the baby as she had a bath, being taken care of, not worrying about what needed doing in the house – she said, 'it

## POSTPARTUM PLAN FOR A POSITIVE FOURTH TRIMESTER WITH YOUR BABY

- How am I going to ensure that I have the time and space to recover from giving birth? What can I put into place now to help?
- How do I feel about visitors in the immediate postnatal period? What are my limits? Who am I comfortable with seeing? If there are people you want to delay seeing, can you set their expectations before baby is born?
- What am I going to put into place now to help me with feeding and how will I ensure I rest during the day? Who is going to help support me on my feeding journey? What support is available in my area? E.g. lactation consultants, breastfeeding clinics, La Leche League groups or similar, supportive family and friends – or, equally, those who have bottle-fed.
- How am I going to ensure we have enough time in the early days for bonding as a new family? How are we going to make sure we maximise bonding time while my partner is on paternity leave?
- How am I going to create my 'nest'? Have I got places around the house to recuperate in comfortably? I recommend having 'stations' on your sofa and your bed with everything you need handy so that you can settle in and cluster feed!
- How am I going to ensure I eat and drink well in the postnatal period? Can you ask family and friends to bring a meal when they visit? Or ask for Cook vouchers as presents? Or can you prepare freezer meals including easy things for breakfast, e.g. breakfast burritos.
- How are we going to safeguard our mental health? What can we structure in to help with this? For example, a weekly check-in about how you're feeling (with your partner if you have one or with a friend/family member). It is also an idea to be aware of who is around to support you with your mental health – helplines/healthcare professionals/your local mental health service.
- How am I going to factor in self-care? What does self-care look like to me? Practical self-care, e.g. exercise, as well as things that make you feel like yourself and bring you joy. Everyone will be different on this one!

If you have a partner, it might be a good idea to get them involved in your postpartum planning with you – so that expectations are set early.

felt like a break at a hotel'. It reminded me of a conversation I'd had years previously when my friend, Jane, had told me how unexpectedly ending up at her sister's (the builders had not finished work on her house on time) after the birth of her first son had turned into a blessing. She says, 'It was great, they would come home from work and stay up until 1am holding the baby so that me and my husband, Chris, could catch up on some sleep.' Then, finally, a few days ago another friend, who tragically lost her daughter at nine days old, told me she had gone immediately to live with her parents for a month to help her heal. These three women, all fiercely independent, recognised that, in this most vulnerable of moments, what they needed most was to be taken care of. To be mothered. Mothering the mother has gone out of fashion in the Western world, but it still remains a strong instinct. It just depends on whether we have the confidence in our instincts (as well as the relationships and practicalities necessary) to follow this path. I think we need to normalise multi-generational living a bit more in the UK. It seems to be seen as a weakness, oddness, or a sign of socio-economic struggle, when it is a perfectly natural state of affairs elsewhere in the world. The fracturing of our families and communities does little to help a postnatal woman, and this obsession with doing it all ourselves, and 'springing back to normal', is a modern and potentially damaging concept.

Moving back could look different for everyone depending on circumstances. It could mean actually moving in for some weeks or months. It could mean spending a night or two at your parents' (or in-laws, if you've lucked out with some legends!). Or it could mean moving back to where you grew up and living much closer to your folks. One of my sisters said to me 'when you have kids, make sure you're near family'. I didn't understand why pre-kids. Believe me, now I know!

If you decide the concept of confinement or being cared for by a family member or doula just would not suit your personality, circumstances or budget, that's fine. There are plenty of other ways to create an environment in which you can rest and heal better.

Ensure you have your rest and feeding spaces sorted, as suggested in Sophie's postnatal plan above. Make sure these areas have everything you need for hydration and rest, whether that be water bottles, snacks, a basket of books/magazines/e-reader, nipple cream, hand cream, TV remote, phone charger with extra-long lead. Whether you are breastfeeding or not, brand new babies like to sleep on you, so you may find yourself welded to your nest for some time. Have plenty of clean sheets ready for frequent changes as your bodily fluids (and your baby's!) will likely be all over your sheets for weeks. Likewise, have throws and muslins on chairs and sofas. Have enough pillows to support you as you rest and feed. This can include specific feeding pillows, but you needn't fork out for extras if you already have enough pillows and cushions to create a little nest which props you up nicely. If you have had a caesarean you may need to 'roll' out of bed for the first week or so, so try to make sure the side of the bed is free. It is best not to 'crunch' into an upright position whichever way you gave birth, so use whatever you need to get you up (I hitched myself up using the bars on our headrest, but other mums use a dressing gown robe tied around something at the end of the bed to help lever themselves up).

Keep going – you're doing great, Mama.

# CHAPTER 2

# HEALING IN THE EARLY POSTPARTUM PERIOD

In this chapter we look at some of the ways you can help your body heal in the first few days and weeks after giving birth.

## BREATHE

You're thinking I've gone daft now but hear me out. We're a nation of shallow breathers and it is always unhelpful to breathe like this, but it's even more important when we've gone through huge life events and/or trauma to the body. Posture affects how we breathe, but that can come later. You may well be laid up for a little while, so concentrate on taking long deep breaths when you can. A useful exercise might be to think of the breath travelling to different parts of your body (your belly, your back, your ribs, your womb). In addition, practise exhaling when you lift your baby (or anything else!). This breath out on lifting or exertion will help support your core, back and pelvic floor. Do not let that breath 'get stuck' though: breath-holding creates too much intra-abdominal pressure. Remember to keep a flow to your breathing.

## HYDRATE

Drinking water is important. You know that. I know that. Do we do enough of it? Probably not. It's so easy to put yourself and your needs last when the baby arrives, but – if you do ONE THING, do this. Dot water bottles all around the house and give your partner, if you have one, the job of ensuring they are always clean and full of fresh water. If you'll be breastfeeding then you are likely to get very thirsty. But even if you are not breastfeeding, it is important to keep on top of your hydration levels. The generally accepted guideline for the optimum amount of water you should have each day is two litres, which equates to 6–8 glasses. Drinking water will help your body to work optimally to help you heal; it allows nutrients to travel around your body; it increases energy levels; it aids wound healing; it will help you avoid constipation (which can put undue pressure on your bowels and pelvic floor). Also, if you have stitches, drinking enough water will help dilute the urine so it should sting a little less when you wee, as well as protecting against urinary tract infections. Although simple $H_2O$ is probably the best means of hydration, teas, juices, broths and some foods like cucumbers and melons can also contribute. Some cultures suggest that drinking cold water in the postpartum period can be detrimental to healing, although there isn't any scientific evidence, at present, to back that up. Warming liquids can feel more nurturing though, and there is (mostly anecdotal) evidence that they aid digestion – either way it's a good excuse to have a nice brew, if you're so inclined. A lidded, insulated cup or a flask will be a godsend as it'll keep your brew warm. Shout out to the mums who are just microwaving their cuppa for the sixth time today! Don't go nuts with caffeine intake though: as well as being a diuretic (meaning you'll wee more frequently) it is not advised to drink more than 200mg of caffeine (around three mugs of tea) if you're breastfeeding.

## WOUND HEALING

It is really important to ensure that your wound is healing, whether that be a perineal tear, episiotomy or a c-section incision site. If you are wearing a dressing on your c-section, keep it on for as long as they recommend. I had a 'pico' dressing, which wicks away moisture and I really think it helped my wound heal speedily. Keep the scar area clean and dry as much as possible. When you shower, just use water, there's no need for soap, and try to air dry. This is more difficult if you have other children to look after, and some women use a hair dryer on a low setting to dry their scars, but I can't recommend this in case the heat causes you a mischief. Most tears are first or second-degree tears, which means some skin and some muscle. If you had a third- or fourth-degree perineal tear (tearing of the outer and/or inner anal sphincter muscle respectively), or a button-hole tear, then please read the latest guidance on aftercare, which should be available on the Royal College of Obstetricians and Gynaecologists (RCOG) website and also via the MASIC (Mothers with Anal Sphincter Injuries in Childhood) Foundation. Do ensure you dab not wipe after urinating and that you move from front to back. Be aware of any possible breakdown of the stitches, and any oozing, pus or foul smell. Burst stitches are rare but can happen. If it happens to you – get the wound seen to, to prevent infection and worsening pain. To ease general pain, a common recommendation is to spritz a maxi pad with some alcohol-free witch hazel and freeze it, putting it in your pants to relieve pain and inflammation. Some women also put some aloe vera on their 'padsicles'. Make sure you let it thaw for a couple of minutes before using so it doesn't cause more discomfort!

## REST

I'm going to level with you. Sleep might not come easy. Whether it's your environment, an unsettled or hungry baby or an overactive mind (hypervigilance can be a sign of both birth trauma and postnatal mental health issues, so be mindful of this), you may find it difficult to get enough sleep. Stressing about how little sleep you are getting can exacerbate the issue. Stay away from articles warning of the dangers of not getting enough sleep. They seem to be everywhere when you are in the trenches of sleep deprivation, and they are NOT HELPFUL. These articles almost never reference the impossible situation most parents find themselves in, as babies are not programmed to sleep through the night. Most of us are pretty chronically sleep-deprived in the early days (I am not going to tell you how long my sleep deficit has been going on for, as a little hope goes a long way, and every child is different!) Don't despair, rest can be *almost* as effective as sleep.

People will say 'sleep when the baby sleeps', and this is a BRILLIANT IDEA, but for me it was never more than a brilliant idea as it only happened rarely. I didn't rest as much as I should have, or could have, with my first baby. With my second, I did try to carve out little bits of time for me and listened to a 'yoga nidra'* track on my

---

* Yoga Nidra is not yoga as you might know it. It means 'yogic sleep'. You lie still and fall into a state of conscious deep relaxation while listening to a guided track. I 'found it' when I was pregnant with my second son, via a wonderful practitioner named Uma Dinsmore-Tulli, and it helped enormously with calming me during a very anxious pregnancy.

phone with an eye mask on (and white noise playing so I couldn't hear the bedlam in the rest of the house!). Do try to carve out some time to rest. You might choose to listen to a podcast, take a bath, get out in nature or do some deep breathing. It is hard to find these pockets of time, but if you insist on prioritising these for yourself, you and your family will reap the rewards.

If you are suffering with varicose veins and/or prolapse issues, remember that taking the weight off your feet (and elevating them if it's varicose veins which are bugging you) will help.

## ACCEPT HELP

This directly corresponds with the above. Newborn babies can be extremely demanding, which is hard if you are feeling exhausted and a bit battered. Hopefully, you will have more than a few offers of help. Say 'yes' to all of them. It can feel disempowering, or that you're failing to live up to the 'super mum myth' (and it is a myth!) because you are now relying on others, but people *want* to help, and other mothers particularly know exactly how it feels. If you're lucky to have anyone asking *how* they can help you, tell them: preparing or buying food* for you and the family, doing light chores in the house or holding the baby for you while you nap or shower can all feel like golden tickets in those early days. If you have a partner, let them look after you and, if necessary, tell them how to.*

## GO AT YOUR OWN PACE

I may have mentioned this before. There will be so much well-meaning (and some not so well-meaning!) advice flung your way in the early days. A lot of 'should' – you *should* be up and about; the baby *should* be put down etc etc. The only *should* you need take heed of is that you *should* be comfortable and able to set your own pace. If you're a person who thrives on interaction and 'doing' then that may suit you even in the first few days. Or you may find you swerve the other way and need to hole up and 'nest'. Or you may not want to get out of bed for days, and weeks. This is okay. As long as you're not feeling

---

* The best gift I have ever received is a delivery of Cook frozen ready meals from my good friends Hannah and Neil – who had recently had their first baby too and knew the drill.

wretched or there are any red flags for your mental health (more on this later), then have as many pyjama days as you like/are able. I fell into the latter camp, as I'm sure you can surmise!

## CAESAREAN RELIEF

Firstly, really pay attention to your pain levels and keep on top of your pain relief. Also, overdoing it really can be detrimental as you can pop a stitch (as my friend Helen did by walking too fast too soon after the birth). You can use a tubigrip, or other abdominal support binder, like a 'belly bandit', to help you feel more confident and protect your core after surgery. I didn't use one, as I knew I wouldn't find it comfortable. Make sure your wound is healed and this is not going to irritate it. Also, only wear it for the first few weeks as, after that, the negatives may start to outweigh the benefits. You need your muscles to start engaging and working for themselves again. That said, Sophie Messager extolls the virtues of belly wrapping in her book *Why Postnatal Recovery Matters*, so – were I to have my time again, I would look into this more.

## PHONE USE

Hmmm, I am not going to get all preachy here. Your phone can be a lifeline in those early days. As well as allowing you to contact friends and family, there are a wide range of supportive and nurturing forums online. However, I know from experience how tempting it can be to sit and scroll, scroll, scroll through the night feeds. This is not conducive to rest. The blue light emitted by your mobile phone screen restrains the production of melatonin, the hormone that controls your sleep-wake cycle (aka circadian rhythm), which can make it even more difficult to fall asleep once the baby settles. Try to be aware of your posture when using your phone at this time as well; it can be too easy to put unnecessary pressure on your neck and spine. If you're able to, sit upright with the phone at eye level and use both your hands – this should help. Also adopt the habit of micro breaks from your phone where you tuck your chin under so that you can recognise the undue pressure you're using tilting your head forward or down to read/scroll – and roll your shoulders back. If you're not keen to abstain from using your phone, then you may want to think about changing your phone settings to limit blue light or invest in some blue light filtering glasses. My advice would be – seek balance. See if being more sparing with your use of your phone/social media has a positive impact on you, but don't chastise yourself if you spend your 3am shifts scrolling, scrolling, scrolling. We all do it! If you message another new mum at 3am, you'll likely get a ping back, which can make you feel less alone.

## TALK

Repressed emotion and worry will show up in your body in other ways. Talking, whether with family or friends (old or new), or health professionals, can help you process feelings around the birth and the transition to motherhood. The people you talk to should make you feel listened to and understood. If you're not getting that from people already in your circle, then it might be time to look elsewhere. There is nothing quite like the bonds you make with other women as you enter motherhood. It's like arriving on a different planet together, or – perhaps for some of us – like soldiers coming off the battlefield. I really don't think there's anything like friendship forged in the fiery furnace (try saying that after a few drinks) of the postpartum days. There is a shared understanding, and you not only go through the milestones of your babies' development at the same time, but you also go through healing milestones together. They may be new relationships, but you'd be surprised how quickly you become aware of the details of your new friend's perineum and other sore spots! The landing strip of new motherhood often accelerates intimacy and helps establish strong bonds. A friend's (in her late 30s) parents are still close with the friends they made at NCT* (National Childbirth Trust) sessions. That said, you may not find your tribe immediately. And don't feel bad if you don't gel with other new mums from the off, keep looking. Mothers are not just one homogenous lump – we are all still individuals. I recognise that being open about physical or emotional issues postpartum can be particularly difficult for some women, whether due to cultural norms, personality or upbringing. This can be

* Many people think that NCT classes are beyond their budget, but the Trust offers a sliding scale of payments. There are now also many alternatives, like Sophie Hiscock's 'The Village Midwife' antenatal groups or Tinuke Awe's 'Mums and Tea' online and IRL (in real life) community.

where forums (where you can remain anonymous if you want) like Netmums and Mumsnet really come into their own.

## EAT WELL

This can be harder than we imagine in those early days (or, in fact, whenever you have full on days of child rearing... Lockdown 2020, anyone?). It is a good idea to prep for this time in advance if you can, by stocking your freezer with batch-cooked food. I made some bone broth for my postpartum period as I had read about its healing properties, and many traditional 'confinement' ideas revolve around warming foods. Having broths, soups packed with veggies and protein, and filling meals such as cottage pies, mild curries and meaty pasta sauces ready to go will help enormously to keep you sated and nourished. When I spoke with nutritionist Jo Sharp, I asked her about a shocking statement I had heard, 'you have the microbiome of a diseased person after pregnancy'. Jo said that the evidence looking into changes in the maternal microbiome during gestation is limited. 'What we do know is that the microbiome can influence the baby's health (e.g. infant birth weight) and overall health of the pregnancy.' While looking for evidence for the anecdote about disease (I couldn't find a paper to corroborate the statement, but I can totally see how this could come about), I fell down a microbiome rabbit hole for several hours. If you're interested in this, like I was, you can find tons of stuff online, with particularly trusted sources on PubMed (an archive of biomedical literature). It is an area of significant research at the moment, but in a (prebiotic walnut) nutshell: your microbiome is trillions of microbiotic cells (bacteria, viruses and fungi) that live in your body: primarily bacteria in your gut. Bacteria get a bad rap, but we need them and there is a difference between 'good bacteria' and 'bad bacteria'. Our gut bacteria help digest our food, regulate our immune system, protect against other bacteria that cause disease, and help produce essential vitamins and hormones. There are also developing theories on how your gut and brain are linked. Indeed, your gut is likened to a 'second brain' and problems in your gut can manifest in mood and energy issues, among others. Jo says, 'A mother's digestive and vaginal microbiome is a reflection of her overall health and as a consequence, the baby's too. With data showing that microbiome diversity is low on a population level and that it affects fertility and pregnancy, we can anticipate that a healthy microbiome will have a positive overall impact, while low diversity will have the opposite.'

You will likely crave sugary snacks in the postpartum period (or, if you're me, for life) but these are an adversary for your microbiome. Boooo! Sorry. Sugary snacks are normally easy to grab and consume 'on the go'. They will likely give you an immediate (but short-lived) boost and you will probably feel like you deserve them because you're working so hard. I am NOT going to tell you to deprive yourself. I love my chocolate and I would pretty much stop reading now if someone was telling me I couldn't have a Wispa. That said, it's worth knowing that if you constantly eat refined sugar then your microbiome can change to crave more sugar and it becomes a vicious circle.

I asked Jo for her advice on what a new mum should ideally try to eat. Firstly, Jo stressed the importance of eating enough protein to help healing. This was something I managed at dinner times (when, as a meat eater, I would have a 'hearty' meal), but I struggled at other mealtimes, as I needed something quick, but I didn't want to eat too much processed meat, like ham. Jo advised having boiled eggs to hand in the fridge to help keep up your protein intake throughout the day. If you are vegan, you could try hummus or nut butter on wholewheat crackers. To help with your gut health, try eating a wide variety of food. Jo explained that the microbiome loves diversity, so, if possible, eat foods of different colours, textures and flavours. When I was thinking of the 'ideal' plate of diverse food and what I would actually have to hand/be able to manage in those very early days (especially when my husband went back to work, and I was flying solo) these pictures were very different. So, this is my easy-peasy-lemon squeezy idea for a lunch time: boiled egg (if possible, get partner to peel it the night before!); wholegrain toast with peanut butter; apple; carrot sticks and a dip like guacamole or hummus. According to The British Nutrition Foundation, we should be aiming for around 45g of protein a day (equivalent to about two portions of meat, fish, nuts or tofu per day) in normal times, but will likely need more if we are pregnant or breastfeeding. The Mother and Child Health and Education Trust states, 'To support lactation and maintain maternal reserves, most mothers in developing countries will need to eat about 500 additional kilocalories every day (an increase of 20 percent to 25 percent over the usual intake before pregnancy). Well-nourished mothers who gain enough weight during pregnancy need less because they can use body fat and other stores accumulated during pregnancy.' They go on to say, 'Community and household members should be informed of the importance of making additional food available to women before they become pregnant, during pregnancy and lactation, and during the recuperative interval when the mother is neither pregnant nor lactating. Making more food available to mothers is even more important in societies with cultural restrictions on women's diets'. So there you go: your community, family and partner should be feeding you up nicely.

If you like a smoothie, and have a blender, then these can be a good option for fruit and vegetable intake, but you need to include protein otherwise it will spike your blood sugar levels, and those that keep the pulp in rather than just creating a juice will ensure you are retaining the fibre. To ensure enough balance in a smoothie, Jo suggests two pieces of veg, one piece of fruit and some hemp or flax seeds. If you do not have a blender, or don't like smoothies (I am not a huge fan myself) then you could spread some peanut or almond butter on an apple or banana and have a handful of sesame or sunflower seeds. Most supermarkets sell a variety of seeds alongside their nuts or in the baking section. Any seeds will do, so sesame or poppy can also be used. When I spoke with colorectal surgeon Julie Cornish, she was adamant that postnatal women should ensure enough fibre in their diet, as well as staying hydrated. This will help ensure that your stools are soft and bulky enough to pass easily and quickly, which will avoid constipation. You should be aiming for 30g of fibre per day, which you will easily manage if you are getting your 5–10 vegetables and fruit a day as well as including beans, chickpeas, lentils, wholemeal bread, oats and so on in your diet every day. You can also take fibre as a supplement, with something made of chicory root or fybogel/ psyllium husk – just ask your local pharmacy or health food shop. Eva Johnson, a nutritionist, notes that you should aim to get the fibre from your diet rather than supplementing – although those with some gastrointestinal issues (such as IBS – people who may be on a 'low FODMAP diet'[6]) may need to use a supplement as a short-term measure. She also struck a note of caution on including weight measurements of food: we do not want to encourage this as it can lead to obsessive and restrictive eating habits. A portion of protein is roughly the size of your hand and there is no need to weigh anything – use your hunger and full feelings as your guide. Obviously, sometimes thirst can feel like hunger, so you can try to drink a cup of tea or a glass of water before a meal if you want.

Doula Laura Rice also gave some excellent suggestions for postpartum nutrition: 'Eat anything that helps with digestion, as the last thing you want to be is constipated. So, anything with fibre that is also gentle on the digestive system. What do you feel like you want to eat when you are under the weather – what brings you that nice feeling? Something warm, comforting and objectively good for you at the same time.' She is also an advocate for planning all this in advance – particularly your first meal after the birth. 'You don't want it to be a cheese sandwich from the hospital trolley. Think about looking after yourself, so you can look after the baby.' Laura provides a delicious and nutritious postpartum menu for her clients which I share some of, with permission, below – to give you some inspiration. I'm salivating looking at it!

- African peanut stew
- Beef and vegetable casserole
- Chicken and vegetable casserole
- White miso ramen
- Tomato and lentil ragu with pasta
- Lemon, tomato and cardamom dhal
- Chicken korma chilli
- Thai baked sweet potatoes
- Apple pie oatmeal (delicious breakfast)

## SUPPLEMENTATION

Firstly, the government advises taking a Vitamin D supplement throughout the autumn and winter as we cannot get enough from sunlight and diet during these months. The two nutritionists I spoke to for this book were clear that we should be aiming for enough balance in our diet to fulfil our vitamin and mineral needs. However, I KNOW first-hand that this can be extremely tricky during the best of times, let alone when you are catapulted into new motherhood and just going to the loo can seem like a mammoth undertaking. So, what would *they* take if they needed to top up vitamin levels? Eva was keen to point out that it's worth doing your own research and making sure that the vitamin companies are doing the research into their ingredients that shows their credentials. Both Eva and Jo cited Viridian and BioCare as decent brands. Personally, I am a fan of Wild Nutrition who do specialist pre/postnatal supplements, which I truly believe saved me in the early days with baby number two. Both nutritionists also stressed the need for omega-3 (a 'fatty acid') postpartum, and if you are unable to get this through oily fish or nuts and seeds, then supplementing would be advisable. Midwife Sundas Khalid passed on to me the most wonderful family recipe for 'Panjeeri', which is a traditional South Asian food used to help support women in the postpartum period, which is bursting with nuts and seeds. See the back of the book for the recipe.

Jo Sharp knows that, without holistic and focused support on providing you optimal nutrition, you will be unlikely to be able to meet all of your nutritional needs in the early days postpartum. She has advised that you keep taking your prenatal supplement throughout 'the fourth trimester', but that supplements are not 'a magic bullet but a safety net'.

## PERSONAL HYGIENE

Never in a million years did I think my personal hygiene would plummet to the levels that it did postpartum. Some days, I would not be able to recall when I last had a shower. Some days, I didn't manage to brush my teeth. This should not be the case, obviously. We should have our village there to help us to look after ourselves, but modern living doesn't tend to allow for this. Again, I would implore you to accept offers of help so that you may be able to tend to yourself. Wound care is particularly important if you have had a caesarean or perineal tear. It is best to gently rinse clean water (soap suds can wash down from the rest of your body) over the wound a few times a day and allow to air dry if possible. If you notice any itching, inflamed, red or discoloured skin, pus or offensive smell – then you need to get your wound checked. Your midwife should keep an eye on any stitches to ensure healing is going well. If they don't – then ask them to. Please don't feel embarrassed. They have seen it all and it is part of their remit to ensure you are healing properly. If you had an abdominal birth, then your dressing might need changing and will come off within a few days to allow air to circulate. If you have a 'pico dressing' then this stays on a bit longer. Germs love warm, dark, moist areas – so, although it can be daunting to have the dressing removed, it is best for healing. This should be uncomfortable rather than painful.

*Brush your teeth.* And floss. Baby can sit in a bouncer and watch you doing it (better than TV). Good oral health impacts your overall health and you also don't want your breath smelling like a dead badger.

## WHAT TO WEAR

- **Pyjamas.** For six weeks. I'm only half-joking. Wearing night clothes will signal that no one should expect anything from you, and you can retire to bed at any point in the day. Seriously, wear whatever you want, but you'll likely find button down tops, stretchy bras, big knickers and stretchy trousers very comfortable in those first few weeks.
- **Compression socks.** If you had a c-section, or other surgery (some people need surgery/anaesthesia for more complex perineal stitching or if there is retained placenta), or a significant bleed (PPH), you may be told to wear compression socks. Wearing these helps avoid blood clots in your legs (you may also have heparin injections to prevent these clots), which can lead to deep vein thrombosis (DVT). DVT is when your calf would swell and be hot, tight and red/discoloured; this can be a dangerous condition as clots can travel to the lungs. Compression socks are not very comfy, but it is imperative that you wear them as much as possible.
- If breastfeeding, you don't need to spend loads on special bras and tops, or modesty capes. The one-up-one-down trick is very simple. You wear a stretchy vest top under whatever t-shirt or jumper you want and just pull up the jumper and stretch down the vest under your boob. Stretchy bras can also take the place of expensive

breastfeeding bras, if you don't need the extra support.

- **Tummy support.** You may feel that you want to use a 'binder' or support wear for your tummy, especially if you had a c-section. Some women feel very vulnerable around their tummy area in the first few days and weeks as the muscles have been so stretched, or because of surgery. While long-term use of such garments is not recommended, as the idea is that your muscles start to reactivate and work to support you, they can be reassuring and helpful in the beginning. Don't use anything that is uncomfortable or unnecessarily restrictive and avoid 'waist-trainers' or corset-type pieces as these are not proven to be helpful, and may actually make things worse. Two 'types' of garment that are usually recommended are a 'tubigrip' or a 'belly bandit'. They should sit from just under your bra to just over your hips and they should cover your c-section scar. Personally, I couldn't bear the thought of putting anything over my scar and dressing, so I can't recommend from that perspective – but reviews show that they help women feel more supported and they believe it helps 'train' muscles back into place.

- **Good shoes.** I am not going to tell you never to wear heels again. In the immediate postpartum it's not likely you'll feel much like it anyway, but at least for those initial weeks give your body a fighting chance of recovering decent posture by going for something supportive and without any kind of large heel. Osteopath Gemma Dawson recommends supportive trainers or boots for helping your feet to readjust and to ensure proper weight distribution around the body. Wearing heels shifts your weight forward, something you have already been doing in pregnancy, but it also may cause your back to hyperextend backwards for balance and this will take you out of alignment. After already being out of alignment for months during pregnancy, now is a good time to try and practise better posture with your pelvis in a 'neutral' position (neither tipped forwards nor backwards). Additionally, wearing heels a lot can shorten muscles, which can exacerbate hip and back problems. Flip-flops and other floppy, unsupportive shoes are not great either.

## THE FIRST SIX WEEKS

It's six weeks after another human exited your body – woo hoo, time to zip up your old jeans, put your disco dancing shoes on and go partay. No? I don't bloody (pun intended) blame you. There is an accepted view that six weeks postpartum is when you should be back to 'your old self' and resuming your 'normal activity'. Inexplicably, this can mean many of us that were otherwise previously averse to exercise suddenly donning funky athleisure wear and going to a park to be shouted out as we squat and plank with 11 other bewildered, red-faced mothers. Although some things should have 'calmed down' by six weeks after the birth (blood loss, swelling and so on) – the six week 'marker' is a bit of an arbitrary milestone. It is a hangover from when maternal mortality rates were very high, as a large percentage of mothers may not have even lasted to six weeks. While maternal mortality is thankfully very low in the West, we still have a little way to go to improve these figures, including paying particular attention to the higher rates of mortality in black and ethnic minority communities. More on this later.

A maternal postnatal check has to happen at some point, but there is no magic switch at six weeks which means you are no longer as 'postnatal' as you were at, say, five weeks or will be at 10 weeks. There is, therefore, no reason not to go to your GP, midwife or health visitor earlier with any queries or worries about your health. If you need to see a GP at two weeks postpartum, then book in to see them; there is no reason to wait until this 'six-week finishing line'. Equally, if you felt fine at six weeks postpartum or, if, like me, you were still in a 'fug' at this point and didn't really actively participate in the discussion around your health, then you can book to see your GP much later on about 'postnatal' issues. They really don't just surface at six weeks and then disappear; it isn't as simple as that.

## THE SIX-WEEK CHECK – WHAT TO ASK FOR AND HELPING YOUR GP TO HELP YOU

In 2018 myself and other campaigners and groups called on government and policymakers to reinstate funding which had been 'pulled' for the maternal postnatal check. For around a decade GPs did not have it in their contract to provide a postnatal check for mothers.

To their credit, many still did it – tagging it on to the 6–8 week check for the baby. However, this likely made the majority of appointments feel rushed and positioning your health as an 'add on' really doesn't cut it. I'll say it again for those at the back – YOU are important. In the five years between having my first son and my second, I can't say that there have been great leaps forward in assessing women at the postnatal check – for either physical or mental health issues, unfortunately. This is the perfect moment to 'catch' women who are struggling and also to prepare women for the road ahead. With time, hopefully this service will improve.

When you go and see your GP, try, if you can, to leave the baby with your partner or a trusted friend/family member (even if it means they are there in the waiting room) so that you can really focus on *you*. Despite my incessant drum-beating on all things postpartum and self-care, I still managed to rush through my own 6–8 week check as my baby was crying and I felt desperate to just get home. This was a mistake. I should have asked for my caesarean stitches to be checked and also for the women's health physiotherapy referral that I knew I was entitled to.

I hope you get a great GP who is genned up on postnatal health and will guide you through your check-up. If not, and you feel uncomfortable in any way, then perhaps call the practice manager and ask to see a different GP.

Your GP will check that your uterus is shrinking back, and they should check your stitches. There are things your GP should *also* ask you, such as how you found the birth, how you are healing, how you are feeling, whether you are experiencing any mood issues and they should talk to you about your bladder and bowel health (weeing, pooing, passing gas), and, finally, about contraception options. If they don't, I have added some prompts below – which hopefully you will feel comfortable using. I am not immune to feeling under-confident around medical professionals, so I do recognise it can be uncomfortable asserting yourself – particularly at this vulnerable time and when some areas are either emotive, embarrassing, or both. If you feel more comfortable with a female doctor, you can request this.

I worked with a fabulous GP, called Dr Stephanie di Giorgio, midwives, colorectal surgeons and a national charity to put together a comprehensive checklist for GPs to go through with postnatal mothers and I know that another pelvic health campaign group worked on something similar. Whether either of these went further, I am not sure, although both GPs I spoke with, Dr Eloise Elphinstone and Dr Meera Sood, did seem to have something along these lines. However, if your GP appointment is more in the realm of 'how is your mood and have you thought about contraception?' – as mine was – then the below prompts may help.

- I found the birth difficult, is there a debrief service you can signpost me to?
- I haven't been feeling myself. I think I need to talk to someone about the birth/my mood/intrusive thoughts. Can you refer me?
- I am not sure whether I am exhausted or depressed. Is there someone I can speak to, to get more clarity on my feelings?
- I'm struggling with sleep; I watch my baby all night instead of sleeping. This doesn't feel normal.
- I'd feel reassured if someone could check my stitches/my scar.
- I'm struggling with breastfeeding; can you signpost me to more breastfeeding support?
- I'm not sure my pain/blood loss is normal.
- I think I might need help with my pelvic floor function. Please refer me to a women's health physiotherapist.
- I don't feel in full control of my bladder/bowels. Please refer me to a women's health physiotherapist.
- Sex is painful. Please refer me to a women's health physiotherapist.
- I'm having back/hip/pelvic pain that is unmanageable. Could you please refer me for physiotherapy or osteopathy?
- Things are not okay at home; I need to speak with someone who can help me.
- I would like to know my options for contraception.

Or, alternatively…

- I am not ready to talk about contraception yet. Could we speak about it at my next appointment?

It can be frustrating that GPs want to talk to you about contraception, often at a time when it's not really top of your list, but do bear in mind that you can be a real Fertile Myrtle just weeks after giving birth, after your ovaries being 'dormant' for so long. It is best to try to give your body a break between pregnancies, even if you are raring to go again. (For more on birth spacing, see p144).

Be wary of the term 'That's normal if you have just had a baby' in response to any physical or mental complaint you have… this is still often used to dismiss women's pain and discomfort. You deserve a full recovery.

# CHAPTER 3

# THE FOURTH TRIMESTER

The first 12 weeks after birth is often referred to as the fourth trimester. This is because it is a period of great transition and change for your baby, and one in which they often like to feel as though they are still in the womb (with lots of warmth and motion from their mother). It is also a period of great transition for the mother, as your body recovers from labour and birth, and everything starts to shift back to a pre-pregnancy state. As well as the involution of the uterus and vagina (which should mean your tummy and vulva/vagina start to look and feel a lot like they did before), internally your organs, which have been squished and moved to make way for the growing baby, should start to migrate back to their natural position.

As you pass the six-week mark, are discharged by your midwife and health visitor, checked over by your GP, and the bleeding and discomfort/pain begins to cease – you will hopefully start to feel more like yourself. I will say again that if you are really *not* feeling yourself, do flag it with your GP or reach out to a trusted mental health charity like PANDAS or Mind (details at the back of the book). They have helplines, which I also list at the back of the book. Body-wise you may be getting a feel for what is healing well and what could do with some more attention.

I honed in on the postpartum details in a huge tome called *Maternal, Fetal and Neonatal Physiology – a clinical perspective* and let me tell you – A LOT happens in those first six–eight weeks. From your hormones going down and up, to your immune system rebooting, your cervix healing and closing, to your gall bladder getting back to business as usual, and your cardiovascular and respiratory systems normalising – and loads in between – it is a time of major internal adjustments for your body. No one else can see this, and you won't feel it, but the activity inside you is immense. It is also worth remembering, as midwife Sophie Hiscock pointed out to me, that you are recovering from an internal wound where the placenta (you know, that WHOLE OTHER ORGAN YOU JUST GREW) breaks away from the uterus. 'Healing to the placental site takes 6–7 weeks', she says, so even if you had a straightforward birth, don't ever feel guilty about putting your feet up.

What else? Well…

## BREASTS

First, this book is a judgement-free zone. If you have made the choice (or had that choice taken from you due to medical reasons) to feed your baby formula, then feel free to skip this section. If you are struggling with not being able to breastfeed, do reach out to a lactation consultant, breastfeeding counsellor or a La Leche League volunteer, as you may find a lot of support. If you are actively looking to stop breastfeeding, with a little manual expression (or lactation suppression drugs if you need them – discuss with your healthcare provider) your breasts will become more comfortable and milk production will cease. Do not empty your breasts if you are doing this as they will simply read this as a cue that you need *more* milk! Do make sure to release milk and look out for any bumps, swelling or redness/discolouration (and fever) though, as these can be signs of mastitis. If you do want to continue breastfeeding, and there are countless benefits for both you and your baby, this section may help you. However, it is not a substitute for in-person advice from a midwife with an expertise in breastfeeding, a lactation consultant, or a book such as Amy Brown's *The Positive Breastfeeding Book*.

I am writing this section during Global Breastfeeding Week. There is a barrage of imagery and messages online. While the rather dogmatic 'breast is best' mantra seems to have quietened, there is still a lot of pressure out there to breastfeed – and a lot of the pictures I am seeing seem to portray a serene and pain-free experience. In fact, I have seen a number of images of beautiful new mothers, in flowing dresses, holding their babies to their breast in corn fields or on the seashore. They are, undoubtedly, beautiful images which show the power and magic of women's bodies. But for a new mum, fresh off the labour ward or piling into bed after giving birth on her bathroom floor, this is more often than not completely unrepresentative of the postpartum period and those early days of establishing breastfeeding. I'd say that the UK breastfeeding rates, as well as online forums and chats with friends, show clearly that the majority of new mothers find breastfeeding hard initially. We do not live in a culture where breastfeeding is part and parcel of everyday life – women are *still* being urged to cover up while feeding (lest they offend someone by, um, using their breasts *for what they are made for*) and women often do not learn what breastfeeding is like first-hand from being around family and community members. Their first experience is often having a midwife wrestle a caterwauling gummy (those gums can hurt!) purple ball of rage on to a scared and shy nipple. Occasionally, like me, you might have someone come and pinch your nipples or attach you, like a heifer, to a hospital-grade double pumping machine. I must've looked so bewildered. In they came, every few hours, to pinch ('hurts, doesn't it?' one healthcare assistant grinned at me while gamely trying to extract a drop of colostrum 'liquid gold' from my poor partially chewed nipple) to milk me, as I sat swollen, sore, bloodied, bruised and slightly shell-shocked. It was not a recipe for success, as you can imagine.

We got there in the end, but my goodness, it was a journey. With both of my boys. The first time was exceptionally tough, and it took a good 12 weeks before it became pain-free. I realise now that more than two weeks of pain, or experiencing severe pain at any point, is not normal. Most lactation consultants and qualified breastfeeding supporters will tell you this. I wish we had been told more about what to expect and that high-quality help was more readily available. Breastfeeding is likely to be a bit painful or uncomfortable at first, but with a good, deep latch this should resolve fairly quickly. The problem is, it can be hard to get that decent latch – for a number of reasons, including having flat nipples, baby having tongue-tie, having very large breasts, a sleepy or jaundiced baby that keeps 'falling off', a baby with a high palate, and so on. Add in sleep deprivation, and possible dehydration if you aren't getting enough fluids, and it's no wonder you're exhausted. It's easy to get into 'bad habits', in which baby is not optimally placed to get enough milk and you are really uncomfortable. It's often at this point that women give up. If you are 'there' right now, know that with a decent lactation consultant or breastfeeding peer support group, things can improve dramatically.

A note on a poor latch: don't be fobbed off by someone, however expert, saying that 'it looks fine'. If it doesn't *feel* fine, then it is an issue. I had midwives, health visitors, and peer supporters telling me the latch looked fine with my first child, even though I was in considerable pain. Even a lactation consultant I hired told me that although my child did have a tongue-tie, I shouldn't 'put him through' getting it snipped as I wasn't in considerable pain. This was despite telling her that I was in so much pain that I could not wear tops when I was at home, and I was in tears most days. Looking back, this makes me fume. My pain was completely disregarded by all but one (crucial!) person. A newly qualified health visitor told me in an urgent, and slightly whispered, phone call to call my GP and *demand a referral to a tongue-tie expert as otherwise you will give up breastfeeding*. She told me this was the only way I'd be seen expediently. And it worked. After the tongue-tie was snipped, it still took another six weeks to become pain-free (partly because we both had to relearn to breastfeed now that my baby had more dexterity with his tongue) and partly because I was also suffering with something called mammary constriction syndrome. But we did get there, and it was lovely, and he nursed until he was 15 months old. I know how all-consuming it can be to try and persevere with breastfeeding when you're in pain, so a note of caution here: do not let this be to the detriment of your mental health. Your baby needs you well more than they need breastmilk. Combination feeding and relactation are both options you can look at in the future if you are really struggling right now.

Here are some of the more common issues you may experience with breastfeeding in the early days:

*Engorgement:* your milk production should start settling within the first two to three weeks and problems with engorgement should be easing within the first week if you are breastfeeding and first two weeks if you are not. If engorgement (overfull, hard and lumpy breasts, with flattened nipples that make it hard to latch your baby on) becomes a problem, you can gently massage your breasts in the shower (warm water helps blood flow to the area) or express some milk, with an electronic or manual pump, to relieve the pressure. Looking at your baby (even a picture on your phone) while expressing can help the milk flow. Be aware not to nearly or fully empty your breast as this will send a signal to produce even more milk! Talk with your midwife about taking a breastfeeding-friendly anti-inflammatory to help relieve pain and discomfort. Warm compresses can help, and also cabbage leaves (yes!). Cabbage leaves seem like an old wives' tale (a term I take some umbrage with anyway, as it has misogynistic overtones. Anyhow, if anyone is going to know about relieving breastfeeding pain, it's going to be those 'old wives' – amirite?), but here's the science bit: amino acids in cabbage leaves apparently help open capillaries to relieve inflammation and let everything flow more easily, which can help relieve engorgement, so you can try popping a couple of clean leaves in your bra for about 20 minutes. I have heard anecdotally from friends and family that this does work.

*Supply issues:* Around 6–8 weeks into breastfeeding your milk supply will likely regulate (become more tailored to the amount your baby needs), which may make you feel like your supply is dwindling. Lactation consultant (and all-round rad woman champion!) Lucy Ruddle explains that this is a point when many women begin to get worried that they are not producing enough milk as they are used to leaking or their breasts feeling heavier. Lucy warns that seemingly 'negative' behaviour from your baby (more fussiness, crying or 'cluster-feeding') can make you feel like your supply is the source of frustration, but she's keen to stress that these are often natural developments, milestones and growth spurts for your baby and that they should re-regulate again. Just keep feeding on demand if you can. Obviously, you are the expert in you and your baby, so if you feel something is amiss, then do get it checked out. A good rule of thumb is to keep an eye on your baby's output: in the first six weeks after birth (after the first week), you should be getting 6–8 wet nappies and 1–2 dirty nappies per 24 hours.

When real 'supply issues' happen there will normally be a good reason – which could be anything from not nursing frequently enough to certain medications/herbs, hormonal issues (including thyroiditis) or even birth control pills. Very rarely, it might be because of 'insufficient glandular tissue', which means there are not enough ducts to produce milk. However, ducts continue to grow through breastfeeding and pregnancy, so if you are planning on having more children, continuing with breastfeeding (or combination feeding) may help you in the future. If you produce no milk whatsoever in the early days, then birth trauma, low blood pressure, blood loss and/or damage to the pituitary gland may be to blame and it might be worth investigating Sheehan's syndrome.

As well as 'too little', there can also be 'too much'. 'Oversupply' is when you produce lots of milk, which is more than your baby needs. It can make you uncomfortable, and the 'let down' can be painful and forceful. Leaking can also become an issue. Symptoms will also likely be reflected in your baby, potentially with green poos, coming on and off the breast and almost 'choking' from the speed of the milk transfer. Oversupply will likely 'calm down' as milk regulates between 6–12 weeks, but if it is causing issues for you and your baby, you could try these techniques suggested by La Leche League:

- Feed lying on your side and allow baby to come off more often. Gravity may help more milk dribble downwards and you can catch it on a muslin or towel.
- Use gentle massage before a feed and breast compressions (see below) during a feed to dislodge the fattier milk from the ducts, which will enable baby to feel full sooner and should gradually lessen/regulate the frequency of feeds.

*Mammary constriction syndrome:* This is a fairly new term which explains what happens when blood vessels constrict and not enough blood gets to your breast tissue and nipples. This can be caused partly because of a shallow latch and can be exacerbated by tension in the body. It can cause nipples to blanch (turn white) both after feeding *and* before, as your body tenses in anticipation of the painful feed. If I hadn't experienced this myself, I'd find this one difficult to believe. But, lo and behold, sometimes, in the early days, when I would take my bra off for the babe to feed, I would witness the end of my nipple going white. As I was also still experiencing pain (AGAIN with number 2!) my new lactation consultant (I ditched the first one, can't think why?!)

advised pectoral massage in the shower and throughout the day – as well as 'shaking my boobs' (a previous career had already given me superb form for this) to get blood (and milk) flowing to the area. The pectoral massage was a quite vigorous rubbing on the side of the breasts and armpit area and also between the breasts. I definitely think it helped.

*Nipple vasospasm:* This is very similar to mammary constriction syndrome in terms of symptoms, as your nipple might turn white as blood flow isn't reaching the extremity. This can be particularly common in women with low body mass index ('thin women') and those who have poor circulation or Raynaud's syndrome. Raynaud's is a rare disorder that affects the arteries, and often causes extremities to go white. Vasospasm of the arteries reduces blood flow to the fingers and toes. Cold temperatures and stress can trigger a Raynaud's 'attack'. It's best to try and keep yourself warm, and especially your breasts and nipples, to avoid this painful condition. Have a warm towel ready to put on you as soon as you get out of the shower, as this is when this condition can feel particularly painful. Merino wool bra tops are also said to help with keeping breasts warm.

*Mastitis:* Mastitis can happen at any time when you're breastfeeding (and rarely, even when you are not). It is characterised by swollen and/or red/discoloured patches on your breast (it is normally one breast) but symptoms can also include: a rash, sore lumps, a temperature and chills, feeling 'flu-ey', breast pain and discharge from the nipple. Mastitis is caused by a blocked milk duct and the best form of treatment, in the first instance, is to continue to feed and offer the affected breast first. You can also try gentle massage toward the nipple and using a warm compress beforehand and a cold compress afterwards (although using something cold if you also suffer with Raynaud's or vasospasm might not be advisable). If you begin to feel more unwell, or the pain and swelling has not cleared within about 10 hours, then you may need antibiotics, so it's best to be seen by your GP.

**Blocked ducts:** You may see or feel a hard lump or tender area (probably wedge-shaped) in one breast. A blocked duct is not mastitis, but it can lead to mastitis, so it is best to try and unblock it before infection can set in. To do so, frequent feeding, for as long as the baby will stay on (and expressing the rest) is usually the best course of action. Lots of fluids are recommended and (anecdotally) using a comb on the breast in the direction of the nipple and/or leaning forward and vigorously shaking your breasts can help 'move milk along'. You can also nurse standing up and over the baby so that you are 'dangling' your breast into their mouth, which might let gravity move your milk down and out. Try not to restrict your breasts with tight-fitting bras either.

**Blebs:** Bleb is such a weird word. In this context, it is a blister that forms on your nipple which is filled with milk. A milk blister. They can be painful. Somehow milk escapes the pore but is trapped by some skin. You can reportedly sometimes get rid of these by rubbing with a warm flannel, using olive oil and making warm compresses and massage (so similar to a blocked duct).

**Let-down reflex:** The let-down reflex is what is happening inside your breast immediately prior to a milk ejection. It can feel like a tingle, or it can be very painful, or you might not notice it at all. If it is very painful, this can be for a number of reasons: a difficult latch (that darned latch!) that means your baby is clamping down rather than suckling; a more than plentiful supply of milk which means the let-down is fast and overwhelming; engorgement; a yeast or bacterial infection; muscle strain, whether during childbirth or from feeding in a sub-optimal position which causes lots of tension across the shoulders, chest and neck. Serena Williams, the global tennis champion, has spoken about how the let-down reflex can happen when you hear your baby cry. Some women feel their breasts tingle, or they get shooting pains when they hear *other* people's babies cry. Amazing creatures, we are. I thought the let-down reflex went away pretty early on (well, it did with my first child) but with my second child it lasted way beyond a year, although, luckily, I never found it particularly uncomfortable.

**D-MER (Dysphoric Milk Ejection Reflex):** This is an emotional response from a physiological occurrence in the body. Basically, when your let-down reflex happens, it is accompanied simultaneously by a drop in mood. This can range from feeling a little bit down to very strong negative feelings including agitation, panic and tearfulness. There is not very much current research on this (colour me shocked) but the authors of one study[7] suggest that the milk ejection reflex causes a sudden (albeit brief) drop in dopamine (a 'neurotransmitter' and one of the 'happy chemicals' in our brain). The mother in the study referenced felt 'helpless, hopeless and worthless' for about 1–2 minutes as the let-down occurred but felt happy and well-bonded with her baby at all other times. Unsurprisingly, for an area that is not yet well-researched (although prevalence is estimated at 9.1%[8]) there is no cure for D-MER, but it is reported that women simply knowing that it is a recognised condition helps somewhat. Distraction can help some mothers and it may be worth investigating medication, or herbal supplements/tonics, which are approved for lactating mothers, with trusted health professionals.

**Feeling touched out:** While straying slightly into psychological territory, I wanted to note something that really stood out in my call with Lucy Ruddle. I asked Lucy whether she came across many mothers who experienced 'nursing aversion' or felt 'touched out'. She was emphatic in her response. Not only 'YES' – a lot do, but she also expressed frustration that this is not more openly talked about. She is clear that women need breaks from breastfeeding. Lucy talked about how – in past times, and still in other cultures – there would be other women around who would hold your baby – or even breastfeed them themselves – to give you a break. Lucy also noted that in the animal kingdom, if a mother has had enough of breastfeeding, she will get up and walk away from her young, take a break and then go back. Lucy isn't suggesting we should abandon our young, and we are both advocates of responsive feeding, but she has a point. Babies are helpless, and they are programmed to want to be next to us all of the time, so their demands are entirely natural. But we have to find ways of ensuring we can do this, while not being detrimental to our own health. We are conditioned to put a baby's needs above our own ALL

OF THE TIME, which can mean we remain sitting in uncomfortable positions, or needing a wee, or simply bone-tired and touched out as we allow our little boob limpets to clamp on and not let up. Lucy said, 'please take breaks when you need them'. I would second this. Nursing aversion is real. My husband and I didn't know what was happening when I experienced what I can only describe as 'extreme claustrophobia' in the very early days (or rather, early hours of the morning) with my firstborn. It was an awful and all-consuming feeling that I just wanted my son *off me*. I felt terrible. No one had mentioned this. And surely, he *needed* food if he was *still* feeding?! My husband suggested I go downstairs to the lounge for a change of scene, which I did… but I took the baby with me. It alleviated the feeling a bit, but what I *should* have done, is to have handed over the baby while I took some time away on my own. It is okay to step away sometimes. Make sure baby is safe, secure (ideally with a loved one, but, if not, then in a safe cot/crib) and knows you are coming back soon; take a few deep breaths, stretch, make a cuppa, go to the toilet – and you will be better placed to continue.

For many people, establishing comfortable breastfeeding is *hard*. To succeed you need grit (but not actually gritting your teeth – the looser the jaw and shoulders the better!) but, above all else, you need HELP! Buckets and buckets of help – from partners (if you have one), from family, from friends, from women who have breastfed themselves (shout out to my friend Caroline, who was basically like a breastfeeding bat-phone for me in the early days), from midwives and health visitors who have *specialist* knowledge, from your community lactation specialists, from peer support groups, from websites and videos,* books and podcasts. In other cultures, there are generational and widespread support networks that help women establish breastfeeding. We don't have that here. Breastfeeding is something YOU do, but think of your breast as the tip of the iceberg: there's a whole support structure that needs to be beneath the surface. As Lucy said to me 'I don't think you can teach yourself to breastfeed'. And if you can't, or don't, or you choose/need to combination feed (when you use both breast and formula) for *whatever* reason, then rest assured you are still doing your best. Your

* Do check out Global Health Media Breastfeeding videos – they are amazing.

child will be nourished and loved and bonded with every bit as much as a breastfed baby. Remember that it is important that you are both well, rested, content, fed. However, it is critical that you feel there is a choice: that you had the opportunity to develop a breastfeeding relationship, if that is what you want. Lucy Ruddle speaks far more eloquently than I can about all things breastmilk related, including some excellent posts about how much more support is necessary for women to be able to breastfeed, as well as lots of information on combination feeding, pumping and relactation (when you begin to breastfeed again after a gap). Do check her out online at www. lucyruddle.co.uk.

After reading all of the above, or going through it yourself, you could be forgiven for thinking it seems like an *utter breast-ache*, but this is far from the whole picture. Some women don't experience any issues establishing breastfeeding at all, and you may be one of them. Furthermore, there are a whole host of positives for both you and your baby. As well as creating a wonderful bonding experience, it improves immunity for your baby and may be protective for long-term health too. For you, it can reduce the risk of certain cancers (breast and ovarian), osteoporosis, cardiovascular disease and diabetes. New studies also (excitingly) indicate that not only might breastfeeding help improve long-term brain health, but it might also protect against early-onset menopause. I am watching this space LIKE A HAWK.

### A note on drugs

Sadly, many doctors are not up to speed about which medications can safely be taken when breastfeeding. If you are prescribed something and told to stop breastfeeding, ask them to research alternatives, or do the work yourself and ask for what you need. *Why Mothers' Medication Matters* by Wendy Jones is a great resource for mothers with existing conditions who might be worried about taking their medication while breastfeeding. LactMed is also excellent for checking if any drugs you are taking are contraindicated for breastfeeding. The Breastfeeding Network also has up-to-date information on medication you can take, (including antidepressants).

## RHINITIS AND ALLERGIES

During pregnancy women often develop 'rhinitis', which is inflammation of the mucous membranes inside the nose. It can lead to a stuffy feeling or symptoms similar to hayfever such as an itchy or runny nose. This delightful addition to the pregnancy package can continue for some weeks after the birth.

If you feel that you are suddenly allergic or intolerant to more things after the birth, this is also not uncommon. There are a few theories about why this happens, but the main reasons seem to be the suppression (and subsequent 'reactivation') of your immune system and the role hormones play. You may find yourself becoming more sensitive to seasonal changes (including pollen), pets, dust mites, mould and, occasionally, some foods. Some mothers report becoming more sensitive to gluten after pregnancy, for example. Some mothers also experience new skin irritations and, if you had PUPPP (pruritic urticarial papules and plaques of pregnancy), which is a skin rash commonly found around your stretch marks, this can continue for several days or even weeks.

## BLEEDING

Bleeding from your vagina should have eased significantly if not stopped altogether by now. A secondary postpartum haemorrhage (significant blood loss) can occur at any point up to 12 weeks, however. This is usually caused by part of the placenta being retained and you will need to return to hospital to ensure there is no infection. Always flag significant blood loss or any changes in smell to your healthcare practitioner. Your period can start at any point postpartum, though it is likely that you will not have a period for at least three months, and longer if you are exclusively breastfeeding.

## TUMMY

You will likely find that your stomach has deflated significantly by 12 weeks, but if you still feel you 'look pregnant', then be reassured – this can be normal. Most women will have a rounder tummy for some time after pregnancy and birth. Your muscles have really stretched and may have separated, and only time and tailored Pilates-style exercise will help the muscles knit back together. If you have a significant diastasis recti (stretching of the connective tissue between your abdominal muscles), you may feel very weak in your core and potentially have back pain too. It can be tempting to get stuck in to 'crunches' and 'planks' to try and get rid of a postpartum belly. Try to resist this and instead focus on good posture, good breathing techniques and gentle stretching to release tension. This can be particularly helpful if you have an 'overhang' from a c-section, as tightness in scar tissue and muscles can pull your body in all sorts of directions. A wonderful, holistic, Pilates instructor I spoke with – Grace Lillywhite of Centred Mums – told me that diastasis recti in particular benefits from lots of release work (including massage), which enables muscles to work back together as tension just pulls the muscles further apart.

## PELVIS AND VAGINA

If you had a vaginal birth, your vagina should be healing well by now and, because of its amazing elastic properties, it should begin to return to a very similar size and function as before. If you have had a bad tear, you may still be experiencing some discomfort, but if this continues beyond 10–12 weeks, or is debilitating in any way, you will need to be checked out to ensure there is no wound breakdown or other issues with healing, including a haematoma (a severe bruise). Although it is rare for stitches to come undone, it can happen if there is an infection or pressure on the stitches from a build-up of blood underneath the skin. The official term is *perineal wound dehiscence*. If this has occurred, you may experience significant pain, new bleeding or a pus-like discharge or, if you hold a mirror between your legs, you may see that the wound has opened. In all cases, you need to contact your health team. You will be advised as to whether they recommend 'expectant management' where they wait and see if the wound heals on its own, or whether you may require more suturing (stitches). If you are unhappy with the recommendation, you can seek a second opinion. Healing of all tears, including the most severe ones, should be well on the way by the end of the 'fourth trimester'; you should feel significantly less pain (if any) and you should feel a good amount of control over your bladder and bowel. Sex (if you feel like it) should not be painful. Any 'heavy' or dragging sensation in the pelvic region, back or vagina can indicate a prolapse of one or more pelvic organs. More information on this later.

## BLADDER AND BOWELS

At three months in, you should now have regained good control over your bladder and bowels. This means you do not leak urine or faeces or pass wind uncontrollably. If you leak when you sneeze, cough, laugh or exert yourself, then it means your pelvic floor may not be working correctly to support you. Common complaints about bladder and bowel function in the postpartum period include urinating more frequently, not being able to 'wait' to go for either a wee or a poo (urge incontinence), leaking urine on exertion (stress incontinence), constipation, obstructed defecation or incomplete urination (a feeling of not 'emptying' properly), and more frequent urinary tract infections (which can be caused by decreased bladder sensation instigated during labour).

## BACK PROBLEMS

Any back pain from pregnancy weight gain and/or anaesthesia should have abated. However, with infant feeding and carrying (not to mention lugging car seats around), your back could be experiencing new pressures. Back pain can also be related to a pelvic organ prolapse or even scar adhesions. Which brings me to…

## SCARS

If you had any kind of stitches, either sunroof (c-section) or hatch-back (er, well, what else should we call the perineum if we're doing euphemisms?!) then you will have accumulated scar tissue. Scar tissue can attach to underlying tissue which can cause pain in the short term, and longer-term issues.

## STRETCH MARKS

After the blur of the first few weeks, you may now have more time to appraise your new body. You may find that the stretch marks that grew with you as you grew your baby are still there. Stretch marks, which are scars that look like stripey marks where your skin has stretched in pregnancy, will mostly be found on your tummy, thighs, breasts and buttocks. They may still be a red, brown, black, pink or purple-ish colour, or they may already be silvery/white. They tend to fade in time but may never disappear. Indeed, claims that creams can eradicate stretch marks are likely balderdash. That said, showing your skin some love with a nourishing cream or oil is definitely not going to do you any harm. I found I lovingly stroked a balm all over my bump while pregnant (top tip: pure shea butter seemed to save me from stretch marks, but everyone is different) and then totally neglected my postpartum tum. I wish I had given it a little pat now and again to say well done! In one of the surveys I did for this book, one mother said it really got on her nerves when people trotted out lines about loving your stretch marks because they are your 'tiger stripes'. 'That's normally said by people with three stretch marks, I'm covered in them', she said. Fair point. YOU get to decide how you feel about your stretch marks, just like the rest of your body.

## NEUROLOGICAL CHANGES AFTER BIRTH

I had a weird feeling, on becoming a new mother, that I was actually a totally different person. This was pretty much immediate for me. It is hard to describe but I remember feeling that I didn't actually recognise the woman in the mirror in the early days. It turns out that this is not as strange as it sounds. Not only had my body changed, but my mind had too. Mind. Blown. Quite literally.

There is significant research on how mammalian brains change during and after pregnancy, but most of this pertains to animals rather than humans. However, in more recent years MRI imaging has shown just how much human mothers' brains are affected in the perinatal period. According to a 2019 research paper it has been established that first-time mothers undergo a symmetrical pattern of extensive grey matter volume reductions across pregnancy, *primarily affecting the anterior and posterior cortical midline and specific sections of the bilateral lateral prefrontal and temporal cortex* (yeah, me neither) which last for at least two years postpartum.[9] So our brains effectively shrink. Grrrrrrrreat! Hold fire though, this is not the problem you may think it is. A similar 'pruning' happens throughout adolescence and it is thought that what is happening is a kind of 'specialisation' of the brain to get you ready for motherhood. You may not be feeling smarter, but studies show that *new mothers exhibit an activation of the empathy and 'Theory of Mind' neural networks*,[10] which are specialised in cognitive social processing. What this basically means is that any grey matter 'shedding' in pregnancy is kind of making way for your brain to morph in a way that enables you to absolutely boss it with your new caregiving role. Not only that, but it also appears that your brain actually grows postpartum. Neuroscientist Pilyoung Kim, an associate professor of psychology at the University of Denver, studies new mothers' brains and her latest study asserts that, 'evidence suggests that neural plasticity, particularly growth, occurs in a wide range of brain regions, each serving important aspects of child caregiving in human mothers during the first few months postpartum'.[11] So you can give a wry smile to anyone who accuses you of having 'mummy brain' – because actually you just got smarter. Your newly 'topiarised' brain will help you ascertain threats and also read non-verbal cues from your infant, infer their needs and respond with empathy to meet these needs. The studies show that your brain continues to morph as you hone your new skills and respond to your infant's changing needs. A pre-eminent research scientist in maternal neurology, Dr Elseline Hoekzema, the Director of Pregnancy and the Brain Lab at Amsterdam University Medical Center, corresponded with me over email to answer some questions. When I asked what happens to the brain in the postpartum period and whether we 'regenerate' any of the lost grey matter (i.e. specific to the site where it was lost), Elseline tells me that initial findings suggest *there is a small reversal of some of the changes that happen in pregnancy* in the postpartum period. The area where they found this reversal was the hippocampus, a key memory area of the brain. She is clear that there is still a lot of work to be done to uncover the full scope of what is happening to the maternal brain. Although she knows that 'losing a bit of brain' might sound negative to us, it is comparable with how adolescent brains become refined, and also 'we found that the volume losses in a mother's brain during pregnancy are related to a mother's stronger brain response to her baby after birth'. Meaning that the more brainy-bits you lose, the stronger your mother-baby bond. Broadly speaking, this is all pretty positive stuff. And not only that, but recent research also shows a positive connection between bearing children and the ageing of the brain. A recent study revealed 'an association between a higher number of previous childbirths and lower white matter brain age.' White matter is your neural highway, where information gets passed between different areas of grey matter within the central nervous system. This study lists several issues with producing definitive conclusions and calls for further research, but it is a comprehensive study that builds on previous research in this area – including a 2005 study on rats which showed how 'parity' (the number of children you give birth to) is 'associated with protective effects on age-related decline in learning, memory, and brain health'. So, big fist-bump to Octomom. This isn't to say you won't experience forgetfulness. You likely will. Hormonal changes, lack of sleep, stress and new priorities will all affect our normal brain function. But there *are* positives to your changing brain anatomy and function. And the science is new, which means more exciting revelations could be on the way!

These findings coincide with a new recognition of the term 'matrescence', first coined in the 1970s by medical anthropologist Dana Raphael, which seeks to explain the significance of how a woman fundamentally changes on becoming a mother. This term gained more traction in recent times, when psychologist Alexandra Sacks wrote an article for the *New York Times*, entitled 'The Birth of a Mother'. She also did a TED talk on matrescence, which went viral (well worth checking out). My goodness, I felt SEEN! Alexandra states that, 'Like adolescence, matrescence describes a developmental transition that is hormonal, physical and emotional'. It is helpful to have a term that encompasses this seismic identity shift, which we can use as a reference point. It can all feel a bit overwhelming, settling into this 'new you'. If it does, have a think back to how adolescence felt and cut yourself some slack. Our bodies, hormones and even our brain have all undergone some serious restructuring. The magnitude of what we undertake to become a mother, notwithstanding the years of struggle that getting pregnant can sometimes entail, is often underplayed. If I had known before about all the shifts, including the neurological changes, I think I would have felt less like an alien in my own body.

When I spoke with consultant psychiatrist Dr Rebecca Moore, who specialises in a holistic approach to perinatal care, she summed up perfectly what a monumental shift childbirth creates: 'Such a unique constellation of events happen in such a short period of time. The physicality of the birth, any subsequent injury or trauma, the huge hormonal shifts, trying to establish feeding – all amidst the physiological and psychological shifts. To do justice to that, we need to recognise all of these shifts and the complex interplay between them.'

More research is ongoing, with Dr Elseline Hoekzema receiving a grant from the European Research Council for further exploration. I have a feeling that there are going to be some really exciting findings in the next few years. Also I will be keeping my eye out for a book that looks at this area more in depth called *The Motherhood Complex* by Melissa Hogenboom.

# CHAPTER 4

# HEALING IN THE FIRST THREE MONTHS POST-BIRTH

**BREATHE BETTER**

Breathing properly is key to lowering stress, increasing energy and aiding pelvic floor and core rehabilitation. Before I started writing this book, I thought 'belly breathing' was what I needed to be aiming for (as this type of breath is sometimes used in yoga, and it does feel relaxing), but I have now learnt that we need to be ensuring our diaphragm (the dome-like muscle under the ribs) is working optimally. Your diaphragm works in tandem with your pelvic floor and, if you begin to breathe more deeply to fill your lungs, and make sure your diaphragm is not 'stuck' and can move up and down freely, you will be encouraging better function for your pelvic floor.

When you get a moment (I know! A moment never transpires, but maybe when you *finally* get baby to sleep in the evening), lie down and put one hand on your tummy and one on your side (ribs, wrapped around to back). As you breathe in, try and envisage your breath travelling into the sides of your body, where your ribs and back are, and a little into your belly. This will ensure your diaphragm is working properly. As you breathe in your diaphragm flattens and lowers and as you breathe out your diaphragm lifts, which lifts the pelvic floor with it. Both breaths are really important for the pelvic floor. The in-breath allows your pelvic floor to relax and lengthen, which is *just as important* as the out-breath, which allows the pelvic floor to contract, and with which you can do your 'upward lift' which constitutes your pelvic floor exercises. If you can, try to set aside a few minutes a day to lie down and concentrate on your breathing. You will not only be increasing the oxygen flow around your body, which helps with healing – and with energy and stress levels – you will also be gently working your core and pelvic floor.

Throughout the day, try to take note of your breathing. If you are lifting your shoulders, chest or belly too much as you breathe, you may be either breathing too shallowly (not allowing enough oxygen in) or belly breathing, which creates too much downward pressure on your pelvic floor. Try and breathe into your whole torso and feel your ribs moving in and out. You won't be able to change a lifetime of breathing habits in one go, but adopting this practice can help you to learn how to optimise your breathing. You can also try to ensure you are not 'holding tension', which can affect how you breathe. Many new mums (me included) wear their shoulders like earrings in the early weeks. Find a time in the day to lift your shoulders to your ears, hold for a count of three and release with a sigh (trust me, this feels good)! Also try to open your mouth really wide and close it like a fish to release tension in your jaw.

In 2018 I helped with a podcast called the Postnatal FAQ, produced by audio producer Abby Hollick, which I highly recommend as a listen during night feeds or walks. On this podcast yoga teacher Victoria Maw talks about a particular breathing practice which sounds simply lovely for the postnatal period. She describes doing this while breastfeeding, but you could do it while bottle-feeding or just lying on the floor next to your baby. You can pretty much do it anywhere, although there is noise involved so you may want to be at home. First, check you are feeling as comfortable as you can. Relax the shoulders and soften the face. Notice your breath. As you inhale let the ribs and belly inflate and as you exhale let it sink and soften. Start making a sound with your breath, as if you are trying to create steam on your bathroom mirror. Then try this with the mouth closed. Try to find this sound on the inhale and exhale. Victoria says. 'This is great if you are feeling exhausted as this gentle sound is like a sonic massage. Try 5–10 repetitions of this type of breath and try to take note of how you feel afterwards.'

## MOVE BETTER

The daily care of a newborn, who turns into a bigger baby and then a toddler and so forth – can be pretty taxing on our bodies. We are moving in ways that we haven't before, and while Pilates, yoga, strength training and other exercise will be beneficial, it is just as important to note how you move on a day-to-day basis. Poor habits and posture can put too much stress and strain on your body.

- When feeding your baby, try to make sure you are sitting upright (or lie comfortably in the 'c-position' if you are breastfeeding lying down). Make sure your feet are flat on the floor. If you are short, like me, you might need cushions behind you and some books or a yoga block to rest your feet on. Try to bring baby to you with supportive pillows so that you are not hunching or straining to hold all their weight yourself. If you had a c-section, a chair with sturdy arm rests to help lever you up after feeds will help.
- When getting in and out of bed, or up from a lying position on the floor, and whether you have had a c-section or not, try to roll on to your side and push yourself up with one arm. This prevents the 'crunching' motion that we are trying to avoid in the early postpartum (this motion can aggravate diastasis recti and create too much downward pressure on your pelvic floor). If you had a c-section, investing in a bed rail to help lever yourself up might help.
- When standing up, try to relax your bum muscles, as they will have been used to tilting forward and gripping during pregnancy, as your weight transferred forward. Try to splay your toes out so that you have a greater surface area, and stability, for your feet.
- Don't go around sucking your tummy in. Many of us have grown up thinking that sucking your belly in equates to good posture, but what it actually does is increase 'intra-abdominal pressure', which stresses the pelvic floor. Let your belly be loose. This will also help you breathe properly. However, if you are lifting then a decent exhale on exertion will help flatten the belly and support the spine.
- If you are using a pram/buggy, try and make sure the handles are up high enough that you don't need to stoop or hunch. If you are using a sling, as well as ensuring the baby is positioned correctly 'high and snug' on your chest and usually in a 'frog-like' position, you should try to keep your posture 'aligned' with hips over ankles and ribs over hips (not thrust forward) and ears over shoulders. Make sure wearing a sling is comfortable for you, as well as baby.
- If you are carrying an older/larger baby, try not to hitch them on one hip (I still do this, as it's second nature, but I KNOW it's

wrong!). Having your baby on one hip twists your spine. Try to carry them in front of you with their legs around your waist and using both of your arms. Also, to avoid lifting that is too heavy in those early days, try to teach your toddlers how to climb up onto your knee for a cuddle, rather than you constantly bending and lifting – as this is a sure-fire way to do yourself a mischief.

- When getting up from the floor, try to form a lunge position (without the actual lunge) first by putting one foot out, with a bent leg and kneeling on the other leg. Push off from you back leg as you breathe out to come up.
- When changing nappies, try to have a change table that is high enough so that you are not stooping. There are A LOT of nappy changes to come.
- Try to stretch hands and wrists if you've been holding your baby for a long time.
- Lying flat on the floor, or with your legs up against the wall, can help your spine realign.

## SLEEP HYGIENE

After the first foggy days or weeks, when your baby is not able to distinguish night from day (and therefore neither have you!) you might, MIGHT be getting a little more sleep now. I hope so. I know how very hard sleep deprivation can be. It affects everything – from your ability to think straight, to your relationships (a friend had a rule that anything said to each other from 8pm–8am was then written off), to how your body feels. If you are practising responsive parenting methods, and you have little support, this can really wear you out. Here are a few tips and tricks to get you through this period.

- **Sleep when the baby sleeps.** OK, during the day this may be completely impossible. Whether it is your only chance to get anything done (a wash, a cuppa, time with older children, some laundry) or you are simply not a napper, it is just not feasible for many women. But you CAN sleep when the baby sleeps at night. It is not unreasonable to go to bed at 6.30pm if it means you can clock up a few more precious hours before the night shift starts in earnest. It's for now, not forever.

- **Share the feeds.** If you are bottle-feeding, you could consider sharing the feeds with your partner if you have one or getting a family member to help you one or two nights a week. It's a slog doing all the night feeds alone and you will function better with support and sleep. If you are breastfeeding, your partner can help with night feeds by bringing the baby to you to feed, then doing nappy changes and resettling while you nod back off. Or maybe they can take the baby to another room for an hour in the early morning while you get a bit more shut-eye.
- **Get natural light on your face early doors.** It helps to reset your circadian rhythm. Bonus points for getting baby into the sun early too as this may help regulate their sleepy times!
- **Fresh sheets.** Not only do they reduce allergens and bacteria, which can affect your sleep and general health, but psychologically – they just FEEL SO GOOD. This is one thing your partner, if you have one, could absolutely do for you. Small amount of effort but huge payoff.
- **Calming night-time routine.** Nick Littlehales, a sleep consultant (this could be my dream job), who has coached professional sports people on how to optimise sleep, has lots of little nuggets and recommendations for better sleep. Some of them are out of our control when tending to mini-beasts, but others are much more attainable. I particularly like the idea of a wind-down ritual. With kids, you can go full pelt all day and just want to flop into bed, but a calming routine can actually set you up for some quality, less disturbed rest. Littlehales recommends starting your ritual an hour and a half before bed. If you are hitting the hay as soon as the baby goes down you may have to speed this up – although, that said, getting baby involved in this might have the added bonus of making them more sleepy too! You can dim the lights, have a warm bath, tidy up loose ends, jot down thoughts or things you need to remember (so they are not playing on your mind in bed), have a light snack (unsalted nuts could be a good choice for the protein and fresh cherries for the melatonin which can aid sleep), go to the toilet and drink your last liquid (preferably water). Also, turn off devices and resist the urge to scroll or watch the news. If you can manage all of this, you are WINNING and setting yourself up for a more relaxing bedtime.
- **Have your baby nearby.** It is recommended that your baby sleeps

in your bedroom for at least the first six months, as this reduces the chances of sudden infant death syndrome (SIDS). I can't recommend co-sleeping (even though I do it and so do millions of other parents all around the world), as there are risks involved and so many variables that can affect safety. Both the Lullaby Trust and BASIS (Baby Sleep Information Source) have information on safe co-sleeping. If this is not for you, having your baby near you, in their crib, at bedtime will not only likely help them regulate their sleeping, as they will be able to sense you are close, but will also mean you don't need to have one ear cocked for a baby monitor and you do not have far to go to manage any night feeds. It also means that you have the option of passing the baby to your partner, if you have one, to help with burping or resettling.

## BREAST CARE

If you are still breastfeeding (well done!), your breasts could probably still do with some TLC.

- **Feed on demand** – this helps drain your breasts so you don't experience blocked ducts which can lead to mastitis, and it also helps regulate your supply so that it matches what your infant needs.
- **Good, deep latch.** It's so important for you to be comfortable feeding, and one of the main ways is ensuring you have a really good latch. Nothing will take the place of good quality, in-person support but a few things to consider include: nose-to-nipple (the babies, not yours!) as this should help the positioning; get as much breast tissue (not just nipple) in their mouth as possible so that your nipple can reach nearer the back of the baby's mouth - this is more comfortable for you and helps baby suckle better; pulling baby gently towards you between their shoulders can help deepen the latch. Your babies chin should be pressed into the breast, not with a gap and their jaw, rather than mouth, should look like it's working.
- **If your breasts still feel full after a feed,** either gently encourage baby to take more (I had a sleepy, jaundiced baby so I had to tickle his ear and run my thumb along the soles of his feet to get him to stir and suckle a bit more) or gently express a little bit (not too much as you will end up with over-supply). Tickling your baby while they are

still breastfeeding might cause them to lose their latch, so try a 'breast compression' instead. A breast compression is when you cup your breast with your thumb on top and other fingers underneath and 'compress' (squish the flesh together) which should elicit more milk transfer, and signal to your baby to carry on suckling. You may need to do this for the rest of the feed if they are particularly sleepy.

- **Air your nipples.** Bugs love warm, moist areas, so try to air dry your nipples after a feed before pulling your top or bra back on.
- **Painful nipples can benefit** from some expressed milk being rubbed on them or a specifically made nipple cream (pure lanolin cream is often a favourite). Remember that pain that is severe or doesn't improve after a couple of weeks is most likely due to a problem with the latch, which a breastfeeding professional should be able to help you rectify.
- **If you are using nipple shields**, nipple shells or reusable pads, it is really important these are clean. Also be aware that moisture on your nipple can cause it to stick to anything you're putting over it, so be careful when you are taking them off!
- **Wash your breasts** in the shower or bath, but do not use soap, just water. You don't need to wash your nipples between feeds. The only caveat to this, is that if you are putting a thrush cream on your nipples (or vinegar, as I half-remember that I might have done!), you obviously need to wash this off first.
- **Have enough comfy bras** to put a clean one on every day. Tight, restrictive bras won't help with circulation if you are experiencing any breastfeeding issues. There are so many more lovely types of nursing bra available now than when I started breastfeeding – but you might not actually need them. You may prefer to go bra-less in a 'secret support' (or no support! – totally up to you!) vest top or just use a 'soft cup' type bra that you can just pull down.

## PELVIC FLOOR EXERCISES

Pelvic floor exercises are *really* important. Regaining strength, flexibility and functionality for your pelvic floor can have a knock-on effect for the rest of your life. So, how do you do them? Firstly, if you are unsure, I would highly recommend seeing a women's health physio to help you locate these muscles and use them optimally. If that is not an option, there are a lot of really good resources online. Two of my favourites are The Pelvic Expert (Heba Shaheed) and Gusset Grippers (Elaine Miller). Both of these women can help you learn both the importance of pelvic floor exercises, and how to do them. Heba Shaheed's site is particularly good if you have sustained a bad tear.

Initially, in the very early days, the easiest way to try and engage muscles which may feel totally shell-shocked, is to imagine your fanjo as a jellyfish as you are breathing in and out, making the smallest motions to lift and release. This should be very gentle and involve no breath-holding, squeezing or bearing down. Grace Lillywhite suggests that any movement, including pelvic floor exercises, which you try in these early days might be best done lying down so that gravity and load-bearing are working with you and not against you.

Pelvic floor exercises are often called 'Kegels' (after Dr Arnold Kegel, who set about proving the efficacy of pelvic floor exercises). Once you are feeling a little stronger, you can use the following as 'cues' to help you:

1.  Breathe in and, as you breathe out, think about holding in gas.
2.  The action should feel like more of a 'lift' than a 'squeeze' and you should not be clenching your bum muscles.
3.  Hold this for 10 seconds (or as long as you can) while still breathing in and out normally.
4.  Breathe in and release the 'hold'. Try and do it slowly and imagine ripples of water on a lake spreading out, which should help you fully release the pelvic floor. Too much tension is as bad as not enough! However, do not bear down or strain to release.
5.  Repeat this for 10 reps, or as many as you can.
6.  Next use the same motion but on the exhale just hold for a millisecond (likened to a little 'flick') before letting go on the exhale.
7.  Repeat these (which work the 'fast-twitch fibres' and will help with continence) 10 times.
8.  Try to build this routine in three times a day – the NHS 'Squeezy' app (developed by women's physio Myra Robson) will help you with this.
9.  Learn 'the knack'. This is similar to the above and is something you do just before you cough or sneeze. It will help you remain

continent even when the pressure from these actions can mean you putting pressure on your pelvic organs.

As well as 'holding in a fart', you can find and test your pelvic floor muscles by stopping your pee mid-stream when you are on the loo (don't do this if you are having any uro-gynaecological problems and do not do it often as you can cause infection). You can then use this to 'cue' your vagina as well as your back passage to fully lift the pelvic floor. These methods for training your pelvic floor have been around for some time, and undoubtedly, done correctly, can help improve strength and tone. However, your pelvic floor is complex, and you are an individual with physiology that is unique to you, along with your childbirth experience. I am wary of 'prescribing' a one-size-fits-all regime. This book goes into some more detail on pelvic issues and the pelvic floor in later chapters, but one theme which is emerging is the need to ensure we are relaxing and releasing the pelvic floor as much as we are lifting, squeezing and strengthening. Any practitioner I spoke to or website I perused, stressed the importance of good breathing technique, posture and relaxation to help the pelvic floor to recover and heal. So, while 'Kegels' absolutely have their place, we should see them as part of the picture – not the whole picture.

## SELF-CARE

Gah, this is a tricky one. I go into a bit more detail on this later on. It can be *really difficult* to enact the self-care we want and need in the fourth trimester. It is important not to completely lose yourself as you are immersed in this new world of motherhood. As well as covering basic hygiene (*when* did having a shower become billed as 'self-care'?!), try and carve out a little time to do things that make you feel happy, healthy and *like you*. As your baby gets bigger, you may find that your partner, or a trusted family member, can have them for an hour while you go to a yoga class, for a massage or a drink with a friend, or read a chapter of a book in the bath. This is not self-indulgent. You cannot give everything of yourself, and it is unreasonable to expect you to do so. It's about finding a balance.

The best form of self-care likely comes in the form of how you are treating yourself. This can come from how you are thinking about yourself and what allowances you are making for yourself during this crazy whirlwind time. In the Postnatal FAQ podcast yogi Victoria Maw talks about practising non-violence towards yourself and also about not heaping more trauma on yourself if you have experienced trauma or difficulty. What this equates to is being kind to yourself, talking about yourself with respect and accepting any new limitations. This can be particularly powerful if you have felt 'let down' by your body as a result of your birth experience. Starting from a place of kindness and acceptance, and not berating yourself, will help create more of a sense of wellbeing.

It can take time to adapt to your new reality. You can show yourself respect by acknowledging that this is your 'matrescence', and encouraging those around you to educate themselves on what this means. Whereas adolescence is well documented and increasingly well understood, matrescence is not. In this void, it might be up to you to produce the framework for what you need. This could look like setting boundaries around visitors, work, or expectations within the home (YOU have had a full day's work with a newborn, even if it looks very different from a full day in an office or other place of work outside the home). Or it could look like managing expectations, learning to say 'no' (to invites, to unsolicited advice, to sex), and reaching out for help. All of this might feel uncomfortable. I am not going to pretend that I felt comfortable asking for help or saying 'no' to things I would normally say 'yes' to. But remember that as well as doing this for you, you are beginning to set a precedent. If women around you (nieces, daughters, friends) see you doing this, it may empower them to do the same when they need to.

## POO BETTER

Yes, you read that right. Constipation is your enemy, and you may need to unlearn some unhelpful toileting habits. I remember years ago going into a toilet in Switzerland and they had a picture of a person stood squat-like on top of the toilet seat with a cross through it. I remember being utterly perplexed. Why would people *do* that? Turns out, these rebel squatters (potentially visiting from different countries) were on to something. Or, rather, we were not, as our 'civilised' toileting habits are actually not optimal for 'successful and easy elimination'. Although studies are inconclusive about adopting different positions for this 'elimination' (having a poo), you'll be hard-pressed to find someone who works in women's health who does not advocate sitting in more of a squat position. There are actual squatting devices (such as 'the squatty potty') that enable you to bring your knees up higher than your hips when on the toilet, which is the desired position, but you could also use things like a child's step or some books. When you are in a seated position (which is how we generally poop in the West), there will be a kink in your colon, but when you squat, or your hips are raised above your knees, this different angle relaxes your puborectalis muscle (a muscle which contracts and relaxes to control the defecation process) and straightens out your colon. Overall, this leads to less straining and a quicker, more thorough… shit. We should not be straining at all on the toilet, and we should feel 'empty' when we have finished. You should also not need to wipe excessively, as this can be a sign of 'obstructed defecation', which may be the result of a prolapsed organ.

To further aid better pooping technique, women's health physio Jenny Constable advises that you lean forward, gently push your tummy out (but do not bear down) and breathe normally. Your inhale helps relax the pelvic floor, so I am guessing that this is as important as the exhale. Some people suggest pretending to blow bubbles so that you create a very natural gentle push sensation. Take your time, but try to go when you have the urge, rather than hanging around on the toilet forever (you might want to give this memo to your husband, or any man in your life!). What your poo looks like is also important. If you google the 'Bristol Stool Chart' you will not be greeted with a hipster furniture website for Pinterest-pinning purposes, but rather a detailed visual of what your poo should look like. Essentially, one is aiming for a smooth sausage and anything that diverges too far in either direction from this indicates poor diet, poor hydration or some type of gastro-intestinal issue. Not having the right type of poo, the 'It Poo', if you will, will likely add to any bottom burdens you are dealing with. The general consensus is that a normal amount of defecation is anything between three times a day and three times a week, but it will be unique to you and your normal bowel habits. Any extreme changes should be noted and flagged. If you are struggling with any of this, it would be a good idea to alert your midwife, GP or women's health physio.

In short:

- Hydrate
- Eat fibre
- Exercise (to get things moving)
- Go when you have the urge
- Raise your knees above your hips
- Lean forward
- Breathe in a relaxed way (pretend to blow bubbles if you're struggling)
- Don't strain!

## POSTURE

Stop slouching! Stand up straight, you'll gain an inch! Pull your tummy in! Shoulders back! I can hear my Mum's directive now, a good 25 years since my teenage self sloped into every room like a morose thundercloud. Hardly any of us are good at posture. We stoop, slouch, hunch or go too far the other way – thrusting out ribs and sucking in belly buttons (we thought this was A GOOD THING...it's not). Pregnancy adds all sorts of weird postural challenges and adaptations, and then as we shapeshift into motherhood, our posture (often the last thing we are thinking about) can become like a sort of cocoon for our baby which, again, is not helpful. Whether you are breastfeeding, bottle-feeding, co-sleeping, baby-wearing, lugging car seats and prams around, lifting a baby in and out of a crib – your body is now constantly meeting new challenges and adapts accordingly. This can mean certain muscles get tight and others get weak. What a Pilates instructor, or physio, will want from you is *alignment* (or, at least, a decent stab at it)! But, what is alignment? Pilates instructor Gemma Dawson describes it as 'a point in which your body is balanced and comfortable, working without discomfort or dysfunction'. What you want to aim for while standing is a 'neutral pelvis' which means your pelvis is neither tilted forwards not backwards (your hips should not be thrust out and nor should your bottom be sticking out – unless you are blessed with a Beyoncé booty of course). You can imagine your pelvis is a bowl of soup and you don't want any tipping out of the front or the back. You should ensure you are not rolling to either the outside or inside of your foot (pronating) and that weight is equally distributed over the whole foot. Now make sure that your ribs feel like they are 'in-line' (stacked over) your hips/pelvis – so not jutting out or collapsed in. Lastly your head should feel like there is a piece of string gently pulling it up from the middle point of your bonce. Your chin should neither be tucked in nor stuck out. If you've followed all of that, then you should be *in alignment*. Try to take note of your posture throughout the day and see if you can correct it.

When feeding your baby, try to ensure they are propped up with pillows and/or rolled-up towels so that you are not hunched over them. Try to make sure both of your feet are flat on the floor and that your bottom is at the back of the chair (stick a pillow behind you, if you need to). Try to ensure your arms are supported so you are not holding tension for long periods of time. Obviously, you will want to look at your gorgeous bundle, but try not to look down constantly as you can strain your neck. Once you are up and about, try to roll your shoulders back and give your neck a little stretch by tilting your ear down toward one shoulder and using the opposite hand to put light pressure on the side of your head to increase the stretch a little. Also, doing the 'restorative' pose below to 'open up' your body after cocooning your infant, will help. You could also look at alternative breastfeeding positions, including lying down on your side, or 'laid-back' breastfeeding: search online for examples.

Correct posture can pay dividends when trying to alleviate musculoskeletal pain, so do try to pay your spine some attention.

## EXERCISE

I've left this until the end on purpose. It's not that I don't think exercise is important. I think it's crucial to recovery, actually. BUT I don't buy in to the 'bounce/snap back' culture for new mums at all. Slow and steady wins the race in this area. That doesn't mean you have to leave it until after the fourth trimester, but please do your research if you're itching to get back in the gym or out pounding the pavements and get solid advice that is really tailored for postpartum bodies.

So many new mums are raring to go on the exercise front. Or, should I say, so many of us have somehow been convinced that there is something wrong with a naturally squidgy postpartum body and want to race headlong in to star jumps and burpees to get back to our 'pre-pregnancy bodies'. I am not going to tell you how to think and feel. I'd be a bit of a hypocrite if I did. What I will suggest is that you are gentle with yourself. Both in terms of how you view your body, and how you treat it. Your body has spent nine months growing a baby, including growing a whole other organ (the placenta) to nourish that baby, and rearranging your other internal organs to make space for that baby. Then it birthed that baby – whether through the rigours of labour and/or abdominal surgery. So, if there is ever a time to cut yourself some slack – then it is now. That said, movement does help blood flow around the body which can aid with healing, which is why you are encouraged to get up and move about as soon as you are able. It can also help you feel better and more energised and will stop muscles getting weaker. I found walking with my newborn incredibly therapeutic in the early days of motherhood. I am fortunate to live by the sea and found the fresh air and stretching my bone-tired limbs very uplifting. It also helped to lull baby to sleep, as I wore him in a sling. Walking helped clear my head and provided gentle exercise. Sling-wearing is not for everyone though – if you have back problems or pain, or a prolapse, it can exacerbate this.

How soon to get back to exercise, and what exercise to do, will be determined by many factors: how fit you were before and during your pregnancy, what type of exercise you normally did, and how your birth went. Most people, after a low-impact birth, could quite easily take up walking, swimming, yoga and Pilates-type exercises in the early months. The key is to start slowly, let your instructor know about your birth and be wary of overstretching as you will still have relaxin (the hormone that loosens your ligaments in pregnancy) in your body. When I spoke with Julie Seal, a creative strategist from the Midlands, who has lived with chronic health problems for years, she pointed out that 'yoga and Pilates' can seem intimidating to some people, particularly those with disabilities or who have not engaged with this type of exercise before. She likes to refer to her movement as 'gentle stretching' and I think she has a really good point. I have dabbled with both yoga and Pilates over the years, and I still get the fear that I'll be the one in the class who cannot contort my body enough or hold a position. Most classes are very inclusive and the instructor will adapt moves to your level and ability, but if you would prefer to do something online, there is now so much available. And if even that is too intimidating, then creating simple stretches that feel good for your body is enough. It's about you beginning to move in ways that feel good and get everything mobile again.

Please do monitor your lochia, as increased flow will signal that you may be overdoing it. I would give any high-impact exercise (including running) a wide berth (ahem) for at least this six-week period and postpartum fitness professionals would advise for a while longer afterwards too. Although the 'official' return to run guidelines say to wait 12 weeks, Pilates instructor Grace Lillywhite suggested six months might be more prudent for many, as it is so important to do a rehab programme first and many people don't manage this in the early days. If you're a real gym bunny or need the endorphins to help with your mental health, I would advise a thorough one-to-one with a women's health physio so that they can tailor advice to you and ensure you won't do yourself any damage. Remember, if it doesn't feel right – don't do it.

I spoke with a woman I found to be an excellent resource in my early postpartum days. Kim Vopni, aka the Vagina Coach, is a personal trainer from Canada with some serious women's health credentials, being trained in restorative health, Pilates, fertility, prenatal, postnatal and a method called hypopressives. She walks the walk as well as talks the talk and has recently shared her experience of prehab and rehab for pelvic surgery. As with all of the women I spoke with for this book, I could have talked for hours with Kim. She was keen to stress that we should not get to the six-week mark and go from 0–60mph. Your pelvic floor and abdominal muscles will be compromised from pregnancy and birth, so it is important to *intentionally reconnect* with these muscles before you start working them. Breathing properly is really important for this, as explained above. Grace Lillywhite was also really clear with me that before any strengthening, you really need to make sure you have done 'release work'. She tells me that it is really hard to strengthen tight, overworked muscles. Below, as well as some very simple exercises to start engaging your core and rebuilding strength, are a few 'release' moves. If you just do these in the first 12 weeks, rest assured, you are doing your body the world of good and creating the right platform on which to build strength.

Initially, I did not understand why the exercises I was being

## RELEASE WORK

(courtesy of Grace Lillywhite)

### Rock to Release

- Lie on your side with both arms extended forwards at chest level with the palms together
- Inhale to rock the ribcage forward while at the same time rocking the pelvis back
- Exhale to rock the ribcage back as you rock the pelvis forward
- Repeat eight times on each side.

### Hip Flexor Release

- Hug your right knee into your chest thinking of letting the leg be heavy and fully relaxed. Try to visualise the thigh bone dropping down into your hip socket to allow the muscles of the hip joint to relax as much as possible.
- Start to circle the leg within the hip socket keeping the sense of the leg being heavy and trying to keep your pelvis relatively still
- Circle the leg in the other direction
- Repeat on the other leg.

### Glute Stretch

- Lying on your back, cross your right ankle over your left knee and hug your left thigh in towards your chest. Hold the stretch for about a minute.
- Repeat on the other side.

In addition to this, you can get either specialist Pilates 'equipment' like a foam roller, resistance bands and spiky balls or you could use a tennis ball or small bouncy ball for running over tight muscles, or under your feet (don't forget those poor soles!), respectively.

recommended were so gentle, repetitive and easy. I found them a bit boring, and I could not see how I was going to get my body back – which, back then, was something that was playing on my mind. Now, I understand the importance of pacing yourself, allowing for healing and building a foundation of core strength. These things will allow you to find the level of activity that is comfortable for you and be the bedrock for your future health and mobility. I also found some of the language that physical health and fitness professionals use confusing. With that in mind, I will be using really basic terminology to explain these exercises.

The exercises below should be safe to do from when your lochia slows down, and your pain reduces. If anything does not feel right, stop. Come back to them when you feel better or flag your concern to your healthcare practitioner. You may need a yoga mat or folded towel to help you feel comfortable and supported.

If you have had a caesarean, you may not be able to get up and down off the floor easily for a while. A suitable bed exercise I found was lying down on my side (when I was able to without it putting too much pressure on my scar) and stretching my top leg out of bed and behind me. Along with foot, ankle and shoulder rolls and pumping my feet up and down to aid circulation, this was all I did for a few weeks.

Yoga is also an absolutely wonderful way of both releasing and building strength. I found Bettina Rae, a yoga teacher with a specialism in fertility, pregnancy and the postpartum, when I was navigating pregnancy loss. Bettina's online tutorials are helpful, nurturing and easy to follow. Two moves which I try to incorporate into any movement routines are below.

### Child's pose

If you have never done this before, you may give an involuntary 'umm' sound as it is so very relaxing and restorative.

- Sit back on your heels with your knees hip-width apart and your palms on your thighs
- Lower your torso toward your thighs while your arms stretch overhead and your forehead and palms rest on the floor
- Rest in this position for as long as is comfortable

- This is also a good position in which to try a few gentle pelvic floor lifts, if you are so inclined

### Restorative posture
- Take either a yoga bolster or three pillows stacked on top of each other
- Sit with the base of your spine against the bolster/pillows
- Bring the soles of your feet together, like you'd sit in a school assembly!
- Lie back on the bolster/pillows and open your arms out to the side
- Sink down and breathe
- You're welcome!

### Clam
- Lie on your side with your knees bent and at a 45-degree angle and your heels together. Your hips should be stacked on top of each other without the top leg pushing forward. Your lower arm should be reaching length ways and supporting your head. You can place your top hand/arm on your top hip.
- Breathe out and gently suck your belly button in toward your spine. This will help engage your core (tummy) and pelvic floor muscles.
- At the same time, raise your top knee, whilst keeping your heels together – this is where the 'clam' name comes from – your legs should be forming a slight diamond space between them. Try to stay in the same position without rocking backwards or forwards. Try not to clench your bottom muscles (glutes).
- As you breathe in, lower your top knee back down.
- Repetitions can start at 6–10 and increase as you feel stronger.

### Bridge
- Lie down on your back and put your feet on the floor so that your knees are bent and pointing up to the ceiling.
- Breathe out and gently suck your belly button in toward your spine. This will help engage your core (tummy) and pelvic floor muscles.
- At the same time push your heels in to the floor and roll your bottom upwards off the floor.
- You will feel your spine lift vertebra by vertebra as you peel up off

the floor to form a 'bridge' shape. Leave your shoulders on the floor and only raise your bottom as far as is comfortable.

- Breathe in and slowly roll back so that the base of your spine and then bottom are the last things to touch the floor.
- Repetitions can start at 6–10 and increase as you feel stronger.

### One-foot raise

- Stand with your weight equally distributed. To try to do this place your feet together and then move your toes away from each other as if you were going to do a ballet plié. Then move your heels to line your feet up under your hips. Check you are not tucking your bottom under nor flaring out your ribs.
- Breathe out and very gently suck your belly button in toward your spine. This will help engage your core (tummy) and pelvic floor muscles.
- At the same time, lift one foot slowly off the floor. At first you may only get it slightly off the floor before you start to wobble. That is fine. Take your time. Balance and strength go hand in hand.
- As you progress, you will be able to lift your knee higher and keep your balance longer.
- If you find these easy, you could try closing your eyes and moving your head side to side, to disrupt your balance. Your body will have to work harder to keep you balanced.
- Breathe in and return your foot to the floor
- Repetitions can start at 6–10 and increase as you feel stronger.

The above three exercises gently engage your core/abdominal and pelvic floor muscles. The reason why it is important to do this type of exercise before you go back to running, or engage in more strenuous exercise, is because the core and pelvic floor stabilise you, keep your pelvic organs held up and protect your back. These exercises also activate the lateral hips and glutes, which are connected through fascia (fascia is part of your internal structure: it is connective tissue that surrounds and holds every organ, blood vessel, bone, nerve fibre and muscle in place. The key word here is 'connective' as it highlights how interconnected different parts of our body are) to the abdominal muscles. This will help begin to heal the abdominal muscles.

Finding time and energy to do any type of exercise in the fourth trimester can be very difficult, so if I could recommend one, I think it would be the one-leg raise. This is because you can do it in the bathroom when you are (hopefully!) alone and the door is locked so no one can bother you and you could also do it while brushing your teeth, as it kills two birds with one stone and is a good 'cue' to allow you to remember to do a very gentle work out. In addition, if you can get 5–10 minutes to lie down with your bottom against the wall and your feet up the wall, this can do you the power of good. This position allows for good blood flow to the pelvis and aids with healing. It is also an excellent way to fully relax the body, as it engages the parasympathetic nervous system – which is what helps you digest food and aids in urination/defecation, saliva production and your libido – among other things. The positive thing about this is that you are doing so much, without doing anything. You're literally activating muscles and nerves that are helping you heal and get strong, while lying down. If you have a little baby, they can lie next to you, and it will still work if you have a curious crawler wriggling all over you too! In the infamous words of a popular sports brand: Just Do It.

Don't let perfect be the enemy of good. Doing a bit of restorative work, a little stretching, and some pelvic floor work every other day is better than not doing anything*at all.


## BOTH TOO MUCH AND NOT ENOUGH

I know, from experience, that this advice – which has been given to me by internet gurus, friends and health practitioners over the years – can simultaneously feel like too much and not enough. Breathing better, standing correctly, drinking water, having a shower and taking a walk. These things should not be insurmountable. But sometimes, in those bleary all-consuming early days, they may seem unachievable. Paradoxically, it can feel like too little in the quest to 'get back to you'. Many women think back to their pre-pregnancy body and selves and want to resurrect that person sharpish. They want to feel the burn and see and feel changes more quickly and radically. I haven't spoken to a single health and fitness professional who thinks that going fast

---

* For yourself, I mean. I know you are doing *everything* for everyone else.

is a good idea in the early months postpartum. These women having nothing to gain from you taking it slow and taking your time, they simply have your best interests at heart.

That pull between wanting to do more, and being unable to even address the basics, is very real. If I am honest, I am still feeling it! I am not yet adequately addressing the basics, but I do know that I need to, to get the right foundation to build on for my long-term health. I am an impatient person. I want to be strong, supple, agile and – yes, a little slimmer – *right now*. But I have work to do and bad habits to address first. Through researching this book, I can see clearly that putting the fundamentals in place with regard to rest, nutrition, releasing tension in my body, and starting with low-impact strengthening will enable me to get to where I want to be without compromising my body in any way. I hope that I have helped make that clear for you too. And given you the permission you need to start small and slow.

# CHAPTER 5

# WHAT NEXT FOR YOUR BODY – YOUR FIRST YEAR POSTPARTUM AND BEYOND

The postpartum period is, generally, thought of as 'the first six weeks after birth', but your body will be reacting to your pregnancy and birth for a lot longer after that. Beyond those first six weeks, and then the fourth trimester – there are more adjustments to be made. Some changes will be welcome, such as your uterus returning to a similar size as pre-pregnancy and your organs 'unsquishing' themselves, but others might be more challenging. Which is why I will reiterate here: take time to listen to your body as you come out of the fourth trimester and flag anything unusual or uncomfortable to your healthcare provider. Take care of yourself! Or, better still, have someone/a village (now there's an idea, why didn't anybody ever come up with that before, wink, wink…) take care of you. You spent nine months building a human, so you can feel okay about taking nine months – or longer – to build yourself back up. In fact, you should perhaps set aside a year (in your head, I mean, as I know very few of us have time to spare!) to dedicate to recovery and healing.

The fourth trimester is a pretty intense stage so hopefully, *hopefully*, you will begin to feel more like yourself coming out of that. You may have adjusted to your new identity more, and you will hopefully be getting more sleep and have a sort of rhythm sorted out with your new baby and new family unit. But there are always curveballs, and the healing process continues for many people. I am writing this section one year postpartum and I have a nagging hip pain that is annoying me. I have just been for some caesarean section scar release to see if that will help – I am still learning too, and I really believe we need to listen to our bodies and find practitioners or resources which can help restore us to optimum health.

The first year of your baby's life is such a whirlwind. They change daily and it can be so tempting to only think about them and their ever-changing needs. Double or triple this if you already have older kids. I had my second baby at the beginning of the UK lockdown during the Covid-19 pandemic, and I was grateful that I had the giant distraction of my two boys – particularly as watching my crumpled-up newborn morph into a real human before our eyes made lockdown feel less like Ground Hog Day. I'm not saying this period was easy, far from it – I'm simply recognising how a baby can, and will, distract you from your healing process. It certainly did me – and I am forever banging on about the importance of postnatal healing!

## HORMONE CHANGES

This is a biggie. I mentioned some of the delightful tricks that our shifting hormone levels can play on us in Chapter 1, and although the biggest change happens directly after the birth it can take months for hormones to 'settle' – and longer if you adopt 'extended' breastfeeding. Prolactin is known as 'the milk hormone' but it also plays a role in your menstrual cycle and your immune system, among countless other things. Prolactin levels are 10–20 times higher after delivery and fall to about 40–50% after the fourth trimester, although the baseline level will rise each time you nurse. Exclusive breastfeeding, and its related prolactin release, was said to be effective contraception back in the day, but I've been on plenty of forums where women have debunked this by having babies much closer together than they would have wished! If you're not ready for another baby, don't rely on your prolactin levels from exclusive breastfeeding (and definitely don't if you're combination feeding). That said, prolactin *does* inhibit the release of the hormones (luteinising and follicle stimulating) that lead you to ovulate, so if you *are* looking to have another baby soon, then exclusive breastfeeding *could potentially* be a bit of a barrier.

You'll be familiar with relaxin from when you were pregnant. I've just read that back and it made me laugh, because if you *weren't* aware that 'relaxin' was the name of a hormone that helps soften ligaments and joints, then you would think I was claiming you spent your pregnancy doing 'Netflix and chill' (the PG version) on the sofa!

I'm not suggesting that. I mean, I hope you were. But I imagine you were doing what most women are doing, which is every-fucking-thing, for everyone, all of the time. Anyhoo, no more 'relaxin' or, indeed, 'relaxing', after baby comes, right? Actually, relaxin levels can remain elevated for anything from 5–12 months after delivery, although how much and for how long does not appear to have been thoroughly researched. The relaxin which circulated around your body during pregnancy, to help loosen ligaments to enable you to grow and birth your baby, can sometimes help create lasting effects within your body such as instability in the pelvis and flatter feet! Health and fitness professionals I spoke with generally seemed to think that your body would not have the same stability in ligaments and joints until after you finish breastfeeding. Women's health physical therapist Marianne Ryan says in her book *Baby Bod* 'Typically, I have seen most women remain "looser" for a few months after they deliver their babies. If they are lactating mothers, they typically remain looser during the entire time they are nursing and for a few months after they wean their child.' Oestrogen levels will also likely be affected for as long as you breastfeed. There is not masses of research on this, but remember to consider that if oestrogen is depleted then you can feel tired, irritable and experience vaginal dryness.

The six-month mark is probably when hormones will start to come back to pre-pregnancy levels, if you are exclusively breastfeeding, according to obstetrician-gynaecologist Susan Loeb-Zeitlin, MD, as this is usually when 'weaning' (starting baby on 'solid' foods') begins and breastfeeding reduces. If you wean off the breast, or reduce breastfeeding, before six months, your hormones will begin to regulate sooner, but try to wean gradually as sudden changes can mean engorgement and low mood related to hormone changes. If your hormones remain 'out of whack' for a long time after birth, or weaning, tell-tale signs might include: chronic fatigue, low libido, weight gain, anxiety and depression, cysts and fibroids, and your period not returning.

Your hormones may also still be being affected by lack of sleep. Sleep deprivation can cause increased cortisol (stress hormone) and ghrelin (hunger hormone) and decreased leptin.[12] Leptin is a hormone that helps you feel full. With these three out of whack, it can be really hard to manage your stress levels and eat healthily – and the two things obviously interplay.

## ARTHRALGIA

Postpartum arthralgia is when you feel pain in your joints. You suddenly start to feel old because your joints are stiff and achy. The good news is that any new joint issues that occur immediately postpartum may be due to falling oestrogen levels, which means that as your hormones start to rebalance, you should start feeling a bit more well-oiled. If you are breastfeeding, oestrogen may be suppressed for longer so this feeling may persist, but should alleviate as breastfeeding regulates and periods return.

Some of you might have felt some joint pain in pregnancy and wrist, hip and knee pain can all continue postnatally, with the latter often caused by the strain of pregnancy weight gain. Sometimes women can feel significant joint pain in their hands and fingers postnatally if they have been clenching their fists or holding on to something really tightly for long periods of time in labour. Dr Iona Thorne, a rheumatologist I spoke to for this book, is keen to do some more research into this common postpartum complaint, but if you search forums (proceed with caution if you are inclined to self-diagnose, as I am!) you will see huge numbers of women complaining of joint pain after birth – particularly in their hands and feet. Reassuringly most of these women say that the pain went away in time, though many also say that they had their vitamin levels checked and made dietary changes. While arthralgia and arthritis are not the same condition, and it seems that postpartum arthralgia is 'self-limiting' (won't last), the Versus Arthritis website has some helpful tips from new mothers on managing life with aching joints, including using baby rockers (chairs or bassinets) so that you have less pressure on wrist and arm joints when rocking babies, and zipped baby clothing to avoid all of those poppers and buttons. Also try to get a change table that is high up enough so that you are not stooping or bending too much for the multiple daily nappy-changes.

## SENSES (SMELL, SIGHT, TASTE)

Studies on changes to smell and taste during pregnancy and beyond tend to be inconclusive, but suggest that some women do experience a wide range of variances to their normal function. The research in this area paints a confusing picture, with some women experiencing increased sensitivity to smells and others reporting much weaker sniff-tastic skills (although the latter *may* be linked to a pretty common condition which is pregnancy and postpartum rhinitis – see p61). One thing is clear: you can definitely experience changes to your olfaction (smell) and gustation (taste) postpartum, although no one really seems to know why. There are hypotheses suggesting that the heightening of these senses is an evolutionary slam-dunk as it would allow women to protect themselves (and their offspring) from being poisoned. This would make sense, but does that make those of us who didn't experience this Darwinian underlings? A 2005 study[13] hypothesised that we may have decreased gustatory function in pregnancy and while breastfeeding to allow us to consume enough electrolytes – which may explain why we are 'drawn to' salty food.

As with so many pregnancy and postnatal symptoms, you can often get a 'clearer' picture from anecdotes women share between themselves. I never did experience a heightened sense of smell during pregnancy or postpartum, nor have an aversion to foods I usually love. The only strong craving I had was for strongly flavoured salt and vinegar crisps. However, online you will find women sharing their stories of changes to their senses – including both heightened and reduced sense of smell postpartum and changes to their tastebuds/ food preferences. Women that I interviewed had often had a changed relationship with coffee (once loving it, now hating it, or the other way around) and one woman suddenly found herself not only able to drink dairy milk (after not being able to tolerate it) but now craving it. If you search online, you will find reams of anecdotes from women whose taste buds and preferences changed in pregnancy – and never went back. From those that now can't stand tea (heaven forfend!) to those that still crave mustard and orange juice (looking at you, Autumn's Mummy's blog) months after birth, it's a veritable rabbit hole of culinary quirkiness. I feel a bit beige as I don't think my tastes have really changed at all.

Almost half of women may experience changes to their eyesight, or dry eyes, during pregnancy, particularly if you have a pre-existing or pregnancy-induced condition such as pre-eclampsia or gestational diabetes. Some of these changes may persist until a few months postpartum, which is why an optometrist may suggest waiting for your eye test until 10–12 weeks postpartum. Hormone changes can affect the shape and thickness of your cornea and mean you may experience dry eyes and/or blurred vision for a number of weeks postpartum. Your prescription may also change in the short term, or permanently, due to changes that occurred during pregnancy. If you experience 'floaters' (where it seems you can see a moving dot) this may be due the strain of pushing during labour.

## YOUR VOICE

If your new karaoke go-to tune suddenly becomes Barry White's 'Can't Get Enough of Your Love, Babe' then you could be one of those women whose voice deepens after pregnancy and childbirth. The research[14] on this is pretty new, and I believe there is more research underway, but I found this nugget completely fascinating. It is suggested that both hormonal and social factors are at play, and that along with becoming deeper, our voices have less variation in tone and therefore become more monotonous. I hypothesise that this could be to do with repeating the same damned phrases ad infinitum: Shoes! Teeth! Stop that! Let go! Leave your brother/dog/nether regions alone!

The original study came about after researchers heard anecdotal evidence of singers' and actors' voices lowering after pregnancy. Initial findings show that 'despite some singers noticing that their voices get lower while pregnant, the big drop actually happens after they give birth.' It is thought that this phenomenon only lasts a year, but testimony on online forums shows that some singers find it difficult to reach their previous higher range for quite some time. Singers are encouraged to rest their voices, if possible, during pregnancy and early postpartum to ensure they are not pushing to reach notes which may be temporarily out of their range.

## NOSE

Allergies are referred to below – and sensory changes above. This teeny tiny section is about how your nose shape and size can change in pregnancy. There is absolutely no research on this that I could find, but not only have I found anecdotal evidence online, but it is also covered in an article (on Girls Aloud star Cheryl's postpartum facial changes) in the *Daily Mail* – so it must be true. Right?

## TEETH

Pregnancy and the postpartum can do odd things to your teeth and gums. Hormonal changes during pregnancy make us more susceptible to gingivitis and periodontitis[15] (gum disease), both of which cause inflammation and bleeding gums. The latter actually causes damage to the tissue, meaning you could be at risk of losing a tooth. There is actually an old adage 'Gain a baby, lose a tooth' but I am pretty sure this is from the days of yore, before oral hygiene progressed to where it is today. However, if you had bad morning sickness during pregnancy, this could have affected your teeth as the acidity can give bacteria an excellent breeding ground. Dental hygienist Lottie Manahan tells me that this acid can really affect tooth enamel, particularly if you vigorously scrubbed your teeth afterwards, as it actually pushes that acid into the teeth. Add to this the hormones related to breastfeeding, and a (likely!) craving for sugary foods and snacking, which can often affect tooth enamel, and the postpartum period can really throw up some oral challenges.

Even if you stay on top of your oral health, you may experience some changes. During pregnancy, your fabulous body enables itself to absorb more calcium from your food, to help create your baby's skeleton, but it may also thieve some calcium from your bones to help with this. Lottie says that calcium is not leached from your teeth. But the loosening of ligaments in pregnancy can cause teeth to move slightly – sometimes meaning they appear 'wonkier' than before. There isn't reams of scientific evidence on this (although a 2020 study on animals did show that tooth movement can increase by 50% postpartum[16]), but there are plenty of anecdotal accounts of both teeth movement and receding gums. So if your smile is looking a bit crooked, or even a bit straighter (yes, this can happen!), or you're looking slightly more Mr Ed than you did before – you are not imagining it.

## TMJ PAIN

Would you quit it with the pain talk woman? Um, no. Just because babies, more often than not, bring untold joy into our lives, our new role as a parent can also often bring anxiety and strains into our life which affect our body. These can manifest as TMJ pain, which means pain related to the temporomandibular joint – which connects your jaw bone to your skull. This can present as jaw pain, stiffness, tooth or ear pain, headaches and even tinnitus. There are a few reasons why this may cause you bother postpartum, including fragmented sleep, teeth grinding (bruxism) which is related to stress, stress responses in the day (hunched shoulders, clenched teeth, furrowed brow – this is my 'resting mum face'), and the general wielding of babies, toddlers, prams and car seats – *plus* doing everything one-handed, from folding a buggy to carrying an infant while cooking dinner. Lastly, this could also be a hangover from extreme jaw-clenching during labour. Hopefully you will have been coached to keep your jaw loose, as it is hypothesised* that the jaw directly correlates with your cervix/ pelvis – therefore a loose jaw helps facilitate a loose pelvis, leading to an easier birth. I recently saw a birthworker post online 'floppy face, floppy fanny', which – as an aide memoire when you're in the birth room – is hard to beat. However, if, like me, you were coached to clench everything and do 'purple pushing' then you may have residual tension in your jaw that needs some attention.

## HAIR

I was inordinately pleased with my pregnancy tresses. It was the first time my hair had actually behaved itself. So I was dismayed when not only did it start to fall out postpartum, but it also behaved in increasingly annoying ways, being dry and difficult to manage. Between about three and six months after the birth, you will likely find that your hair starts shedding alarmingly quickly. This is called telogen effluvium and is the result of a drop in oestrogen. While pregnant, the surge in oestrogen prolongs the growth phase in your hair and you get less shedding than you would normally. Postpartum,

---

* I wasn't able to find a paper to support this, but it is a strongly held belief among birth workers and other body workers. There have been papers on jaw tension translating to pain elsewhere in the body, including the hips.

the hormone drop means this hair begins to shed again. I would pull out large clumps every time I showered and ended up with balding temples (it's a look!). When I spoke with trichologist Sally-Ann Tarver, she said, 'Don't panic. Most cases of hair loss are totally natural and rectify within a year. There will be a lot of change within that first year. Your regrowth may look odd. You may lose hair at your temples as that is the weakest area and you may end up with "horns" or slightly odd sideburns as it grows back'. Hair loss is an entirely normal, though somewhat shocking if you are not expecting it, part of postpartum! That said, if the hair loss is really significant or ongoing (longer than 12 months), it would be worth seeking help from your GP and/or a trichologist. Those of us with diabetes (type one or two) may find a deficiency of B12 vitamin[17] might make us more susceptible to hair loss, so this is definitely worth investigating. Other factors which can affect the absorption of Vitamin B12 (critical for hair health, as well as general brain and nerve function) are having Crohn's disease or pernicious anaemia or being coeliac, and also using proton pump inhibitors[18] (over the counter medication that helps prevent excess stomach acid). People on vegetarian or vegan diets also need to be mindful that they are getting enough vitamin B12.

As well as hair loss, many women experience other significant changes with their hair, whether it be becoming more dry, more curly or changing colour. There were a significant number of women in an article I read in *The Cut* who spoke of a wayward section of curly hair sprouting from the back of their head postpartum. Hair can often become darker after pregnancy, or sometimes regrowth will be grey (yup, I found this. Hello glitter streaks).

## BREASTS

Breastfeeding will affect your hormone levels for as long as you breastfeed for – with oestrogen supressed and prolactin increased until cessation. How much these hormones are increased/decreased will be dependent on how much you breastfeed. For example, I am about to reach sixteen months of breastfeeding and my periods have returned to a fairly normal cycle, which would indicate that my oestrogen levels are normalising. It is thought that relaxin, as well as prolactin, hangs around for as long as you are breastfeeding, but we do not know how much and what type of effects they have.

Many women worry about the consequences effect of breastfeeding, but evidence suggests that age, rapid weight gain and loss (associated with pregnancy) and good old *hormones* are 'to blame' for any sagging. Some women find that their breasts appear smaller after breastfeeding, but some also report them remaining larger. Lactation consultant Lucy Ruddle states that she went up a whole cup size throughout her pregnancies and stayed that way. I am still breastfeeding but I know my breasts were also a cup size larger between pregnancies, even after I'd finished nursing. You may also find your breasts are more lop-sided while you are nursing, as one breast may produce more milk or a baby can have a 'favourite' boob. To avoid this, you can encourage equal feeding on either side but, in real life, most women have slightly different sized breasts anyway. If it persists after weaning, is really significant and bothers you, you could look at padding your bra out on one side with a 'chicken fillet' (does that term give anyone else the screaming ab-dabs? Just me? OK).

It might also be a good time to ask ourselves why pert boobs are so important to us? In a world that still seems to worship youth when it comes to beauty, it would be nice to free up space in our minds by finding more acceptance of our changes, and the beauty in them. That said, if your boobs are getting you down, in more ways than one, it might be a good idea to find a respected bra measurement service and invest in some new underwear that will make you feel good about your body – and fit/support you correctly! Also, anything tight or restrictive against your breasts (so if you're getting back into your old bras, and they no longer fit properly, for example) can cause milk blockages too. Bear in mind that this goes for seatbelts too, if you are now venturing further afield.

As your baby grows and your routine changes, you may find that you are going longer between feeds, due to work, your little one going to childcare or even (hallelujah!) help from relatives. All of this can mean you are more susceptible to mastitis. Your baby might start sleeping for longer stretches at night (mine didn't, but *may the sleep be with you*), so do try to make sure you are managing this by pumping/expressing little bits to relieve pressure.

It may surprise you to hear that your breasts may be a bit achy and even produce milk for some time after you stop breastfeeding. I remember an acquaintance telling me that she squeezed some drops of milk out *two years* after she stopped breastfeeding.* No one really knows why this is, but when I was chatting with Anna Le Grange (lactation consultant and author of *Mindful Breastfeeding*), she told me that in other cultures, grandmothers who have been through menopause sometimes breastfeed their grandchildren years after 'ceasing lactation'. It actually blew my mind. A wonderful book, *Breastfeeding and Human Lactation* by Jan Riordan and Karen Wambach, details how women have used 'wet nurses' throughout history to help with breastfeeding as well as how, in same-sex couples, both women can lactate. We are amazing creatures. I mean, we already knew breasts were bloody amazing, but this is another level. We can breastfeed others' infants, we can breastfeed even if we haven't been pregnant, we can breastfeed years after our chicks have flown the nest, maybe even when we're drawing our pension! If you subscribe to the idea that breastmilk is liquid gold, then you might be thrilled to be able to get your mitts on a little of that 'cure-all' later down the line. If it happens to me, I might run around the house looking for someone with a touch of conjunctivitis or a small graze so I can put it to good use!

## RIBS AND HIPS

The hips don't lie. And neither do the ribs. For someone who already had a somewhat disproportionate ribcage, my 'enhanced' ribcage after pregnancy came as something of a bummer. As most parts of me started to shrink back and I could fit into some of my old wardrobe, my ribs did not and a few really lovely dresses went to my nieces and charity shops. Hormonal shifts enable your body to expand both ribs and hips to make room for your baby. Sometimes, though, these do not return to pre-pregnancy width, which means you may want to hang on to bra extenders and those handy button 'stretchers' for trousers a while longer, while you figure out what is going to go back and what is here to stay.

---

* Once you are a mum, there is no such thing as TMI (too much information).

## NAILS

Finger and toenails are made of the same protein as hair: keratin. It stands to reason, then, that a similar phenomenon may happen to nails as it does with hair. During pregnancy, as you grow lustrous locks, you may see an acceleration in nail growth, or stronger nails. But when your hair falls out, you may also find your nails becoming weaker and more brittle. Some women also find that their nails are actually more brittle during pregnancy, but nails should return to normal within the first year. 'Beau's lines' are horizontal ridges that can appear on nails after stress, illness and – sometimes – pregnancy. They signal where nail growth has 'paused', but should simply grow out. However, there is a small amount of evidence to indicate that they may relate to a thyroid issue.

## MUM THUMB

It's not just you! It is a thing! Its proper medical name is De Quervain's tenosynovitis. Pain and swelling near the base of the thumb, with difficulty pinching or grasping, are the main symptoms. This is caused by inflammation of the 'sheath' that allows tendons to move the thumb. The pain can range from mild to severe, and although papers suggest 1 in 4 mothers get this, physiotherapists estimate that it's more like 90%. The main reason is thought to be the stress put on the tendons by new, repetitive movements associated with caring for a new baby: lifting, carrying, nursing, nappy changing. Scrolling and tapping on your phone (which can happen quite a lot in the first year!) can add strain to an already inflamed area.

## CARPAL TUNNEL SYNDROME

Carpal tunnel syndrome is something that often flares up in pregnancy because of swelling, which irritates the median nerve. Carpal tunnel can cause numbness, tingling, or weakness in your hand. The median nerve runs the length of your arm, goes through a passage in your wrist called the carpal tunnel, and ends in your hand. This is why it can sometimes feel difficult to grip things. I had it with my first pregnancy and luckily it eased almost straight away after the birth, but I know that for some people it can continue into the postpartum period. Water retention, hormones, nursing and how you hold your baby may exacerbate symptoms, but it should resolve within a few weeks or months. Very occasionally the syndrome persists and you may be given a splint to wear and/or some gentle strengthening/relaxing exercises.

## SKIN

My skin was just lovely (for the first time in ages, if not forever) after the birth of my second son. Then it went all crappy and dry and bumpy again. I was not best pleased. Your skin is the biggest organ in your body and often does not escape the effects of pregnancy and postpartum. Whether it be acne, dry skin, stretch marks or a myriad of other 'issues', your skin may take a while to return to your 'normal'. Like hair and nails, skin health can often be an indicator of things going on 'systemically' (under the skin), so if there is something beyond an aesthetic niggle it is worth seeing a dermatologist.

*Melasma.* Melasma (or 'chloasma') is also often called 'the mask of pregnancy', as it is a skin condition which can be brought on by pregnancy (reportedly 50% of us will develop this to a certain degree). Hormonal changes trigger 'melanocytes' which cause brown or greyish patches of pigmentation (colour) to develop, usually on the face, but it can affect other parts of the body exposed to sunlight, like the forearms and chest. Melasma is more common in women of colour and those who tan very quickly, but can occur in anyone. This 'condition' can continue for several months postpartum and so it is wise to use a high-factor sunscreen, as sunlight is a trigger, diligently. It is worth noting that the contraceptive pill can also cause melasma. While there are several 'cures' out there, it seems patience might be the best course of action as a recent paper[19] states 'Patients who seek no treatment and avoid the sun will notice that "the rash" usually disappears in a few months'.

*Cherry angioma.* Another unusual skin change that can hang around after pregnancy, although much less common than melasma, is 'cherry angioma'. These are small red or purple-ish papules that pop up when there's an overgrowth of blood vessels in one area. No surprise that my tummy became dotted with them in pregnancy then! I hadn't paid any attention to them until a midwife poked at them during an examination and said 'Oooh, I had lots of these too.' Black, brown and white women are equally susceptible to them, although they are more noticeable on white skin. Cherry angiomas are harmless and, unlike melasma, probably won't go away but may actually increase with age (quantity, not size). However, sometimes they can bleed with trauma and if you have a sudden proliferation of them then it is always worthwhile getting checked out.

*Moles.* Moles can change during pregnancy, particularly where the skin may have stretched around the abdomen, breasts and hips. If these changes are symmetrical, you have no need to worry but if they are looking very different (multiple colours, asymmetrical, constantly changing or getting very large) you might want to get them looked at.

*Skin tags.* Pointless things. Just little wobbly blobs of tissue and blood vessels. Just one of those pregnancy things that is, like, *why*? But, reassuringly, they are also not anything to worry about (as long as they are not causing you pain) and they often 'fall off' or shrink after pregnancy. Whew. Be gone, pointless blobs. Don't be tempted to pick at them or use hair or thread to tie them off, as you could end up accidently causing an infection.

*Acne.* I weep. Yes, it can be a postpartum thing – as well as a teenage thing, a pregnancy thing and a perimenopausal thing. Hormones, sleep deprivation, stress, poor diet, lack of hydration, suspect hygiene practices (show me a Mum who has *not* just gone for a wet wipe at the end of the day sometimes… Caroline Hirons don't kill me!). All of this can create the most lovely playground for sebum (oil) which can clog pores and lead to breakouts. Also, if you're trying to avoid melasma (above) and have been diligently applying your sunscreen… but then are too damned tired to wash it off, that's some very clogged-up skin. Your pregnancy acne, if you had it, is likely to subside as your hormones settle down, but this can obviously take longer if you breastfeed. Don't let pimply skin put you off breastfeeding though, as with a broader look at your overall health (hydration, sleep, stress levels, self-care) your skin will likely improve over time anyway. If it doesn't, and particularly if you have painful cyst-type spots, you can ask your GP for a referral to a dermatologist.

**Loose skin.** When you are looking at that delightful bump out in front of you, it probably never crosses your mind to think about what happens to all that stretched skin. You may start thinking about how the bump will shrink postpartum, but it can come as a surprise if you're left with some loose skin. If you are suffering with loose skin, then first look at how quickly you are shedding the pregnancy weight. This is another reason why it can pay to go slowly and gently with your recovery, as rapid weight loss can exacerbate loose skin issues. If you lose weight slowly and steadily, your skin can more easily adjust accordingly as it shrinks back. If you lose your postpartum weight very fast, you may be left with excess wrinkly or crepey skin. If you already have this issue, time is still a great healer and with time and hydration skin is likely to regain some of its elasticity.

**Dry skin.** I definitely felt like a reptile after the birth of my first son. The drop in progesterone after the birth can make skin feel dryer, alongside the usual culprits of stress, dehydration (particularly if breastfeeding) and sleep deprivation. You will likely find yourself washing your hands more than usual (especially after all those newborn nappy changes), which can irritate the skin on your hands.

**Stretch marks.** Helloooo, we're still here. Great, settle in then.

**Colours.** Your skin can come up with some pretty different and interesting colour changes throughout pregnancy, some of which disappear postpartum, and some of which hang around.

- **Linea alba** – in most cases, this dark line that develops from your navel to pubic bone (although it can extend higher; even right up to your chest) will disappear after pregnancy, but sometimes it persists.
- **Tits and bits** – your areolae, armpits, nipples and vulval tissue can all darken throughout pregnancy. Again, in some women, this change may be permanent. I was fascinated to find out that your

nipples can darken and look larger to enable your baby to find them and suckle. Magic. 'Hyperpigmentation' (darkening of the skin) in pregnancy is more prevalent in women of colour.

- **Spider veins** (telangiectasias) are a vascular issue, but obviously are visible on the skin. They are dilated or burst blood vessels and they branch out across your skin in red, purple or blue patterns and often occur in pregnancy due to the increase in blood volume. As your blood volume returns to normal, spider veins should become less obvious. These veins are not raised like varicose veins are.
- **Prominent veins on your breasts** are normal, both in pregnancy and beyond (especially if you are breastfeeding). Again this is vascular, due to increased blood flow in the area, and absolutely nothing to worry about.

## TUMMY TROUBLE

It may be that you feel you still look pregnant (I kinda think I always did. I've *always* had a pot belly and have been known to accept a proffered train seat way before I was ever actually pregnant); or you have excess crepey skin where the skin was pulled taut over your bump; or your skin hangs low and jiggly… these are all things that we may contend with after growing a human inside us. And it can be hard to adjust. You may pat your tummy reverently and say 'you were a house and a home, my friend' or you may reach for the control knickers and sometimes have a weep. It really isn't anybody's place to tell you how to feel about your postnatal body. We are bombarded with messages to 'learn to love' our tummies – our pouches, our stretch marks, our scars. Well, I'm here to say it's great if you do, but it's also okay if you don't. The body positivity movement is generally such a force for good, but sometimes it can make us feel worse. We don't need another stick to beat ourselves with. Some mothers love showing off their 'tiger stripes', some decide to have tattoos over and around stretch marks and c-section scars, and others want to keep their tummy under wraps. Every approach is valid.

That said, your abdomen *is* key to your core strength and your overall long-term health. Improving core strength can help improve diastasis recti (when your stomach muscles separate, see below), and can help improve pain symptoms in the body, as well as pelvic issues. In addition, 'fat around the middle' can predispose you to longer-term chronic health issues such as Type 2 diabetes and heart disease,[20] so paying some attention to your tummy is not a bad thing. The fat around the tummy is a mixture of subcutaneous fat (just under the skin, you can pinch this) and visceral fat (lies in the space between organs, you cannot see or feel it). Too much fat, particularly visceral fat, can trigger inflammation. Research is ongoing but it's pretty much accepted that tummy fat triggers inflammation more than fat found stored around buttocks and thighs.

*Belly button.* There's not much science stuff on this (I guess there are more important things in life than whether you are 'an inny' or 'an outy') however, if you were previously an inny and are now an outy, I cannot guarantee it will go back in. However, if the skin around your new outy is tender and there is more of a bulge beneath your belly button, then you may have an umbilical hernia (when part of your intestine bulges through the opening in your abdominal muscles near your belly button) which will need investigating if it is causing you discomfort or pain.

*Diastasis recti.* I had never heard of this before my first birth and had no idea what it meant. I find it mindboggling that we aren't informed at the outset about the changes that can happen to our bodies during pregnancy – and this is a biggie. Diastasis means separation and recti is short for 'recti abdominus' – the 'recti' being a pair of long flat muscles at the front of the abdomen, joining the sternum (the bit under your breasts in the mid-line of your body) to the pubis (the front of the pelvis) and helping you to bend forwards or sideways. The muscles separate along the mid-line of connective tissue, as the uterus grows and pushes them apart, to make room for the baby. Your body is pretty nifty, you know! Doula Suzzie Vehrs describes it as 'when the connective tissue between your abdominals, the linea alba, weakens and stretches out. Imagine the linea alba as a zipper holding the left and right sides of your abdominals together. When zipped-up tight, everything feels right and good. Now imagine someone has undone the zipper that holds the two sides of your abdominal walls together. This is diastasis recti. Your stomach looks different. Your body feels different. Because you are unzipped, you have lost your centre of support, so you move differently'.

Sometimes this will be a small separation, and hardly noticeable, and sometimes it will be very significant. It is reported that 100%[21] of women who reach 35 weeks pregnant will experience some degree of diastasis recti, so it is a very normal part of how your body adapts for pregnancy. How much it affects you seems to be somewhat down to chance, as the study in 2014 (referenced above) showed that your own weight, and the weight of the baby, did not have huge bearing on diastasis at six months postpartum. There is no way that we know of yet, to predict who will experience a large separation and there is no way of preventing it. Up to a third of women will continue to have this gap at 12 months postpartum. Most will not suffer pain or discomfort, but the separation may cause you to feel instability in your core and it can affect how your stomach looks – often contributing to a 'poochy' or domed tummy. A women's health physio is best placed to diagnose diastasis recti, but you can also try to check how long/deep it is yourself by lying on your back, with your knees bent, and walking your hand down the midline of your belly, seeing if the tissue feels hollow or taut. You can then press three fingers just above your belly button as you exhale and gently lift your head. Feel where on your fingers feels hollow or you can push in deep, and where you feel tension from the muscles. This will give you an idea as to how deep and wide the separation is. But don't despair! These separations can, and do, heal. Some heal on their own and others will need help – and even those that don't heal don't mean that you cannot help your stomach muscles and core in other ways. There is ongoing research and work on 'healing' diastasis, but current thinking suggests that even if you do have a significant gap it is more about how much tension your muscles are able to create, and you can actually be more functional with a large DR than someone without one, depending on overall fitness levels.

*C-section 'overhang'.* An aesthetic aspect of a c-section which some mothers struggle with is the 'overhang'. The c-section 'shelf' is an overhang of skin and fat above your scar. For some it is barely noticeable, but for others it is very pronounced, so much so that it feels like a 'flap' (sometimes, annoyingly, called a 'mother's apron') that they need to lift up and wash under. Not everyone gets this, and it does seem somewhat arbitrary as to who does and who doesn't, as it is not always those of us with larger tummies who experience this. I say it's aesthetic, but it's not really solely that, as this extra 'pooch' of skin (and sometimes, fat) can be very uncomfortable, with women unable to find clothes with a waistband that fits properly. Some people can be blasé and unsympathetic about this issue, often brushing it off with 'you're fine and the baby is healthy' comments, but this can be deeply affecting. A c-section support group I am on clearly highlights what an issue the 'overhang/pooch' is for everyone, as there are hundreds, if not thousands, of posts about this, with some mothers really struggling mentally with this change to their bodies.

***Phantom kicks.*** Something else you may not have heard of is 'phantom kicks'. I hadn't and I wondered if a) they'd left someone in there or b) I was going barmy. Neither were the case. Phantom kicks are a thing. The sensations feel like little flutters and kicks in the womb, just like you have in pregnancy. There is no consensus on why this happens, but one theory is that the uterus can take a long time to stop contracting and settle down after giving birth. Other theories include a mother simply being more attuned to every twitch and flicker in her tummy after concentrating so hard on her body during pregnancy, or that she is experiencing a similar phenomenon to the 'phantom limb' syndrome that amputees report. The latter is potentially caused by increased 'innervation of the abdominal region by ongoing foetal movement [...] over the ~40week gestation'[22] which 'rapidly ceases at childbirth' – meaning that you have increased nerve activation during pregnancy which comes to an abrupt stop at birth, leaving your nerves still 'reacting' as if to movement, even though nothing is there. This seems more likely to me, especially after having experienced it myself and it feeling *exactly* like a baby kicking and *not at all* like a rumbly tummy that my silly postpartum brain couldn't differentiate between. According to the survey cited above, although many women will associate these sensations with a positive feeling and nostalgia, some women may find they trigger anxiety – especially those women who have experienced pregnancy or baby loss.

*Scar tissue.* Whether you have a caesarean, perineal or internal scar, you will have some degree of scar tissue. The job of scar tissue is to protect your body by closing a wound as quickly as possible. Physiotherapist Edel McCann, known as 'Physio Mummy' and based in Edinburgh, likens the establishment of scar tissue to 'a spider's web' saying, 'The body will lay down fibre as fast as it can, in whatever way it can'. Fibrous tissue replaces healthy tissue to allow your wounds and incisions to heal. We are not told much about how to help our scars heal, and certainly nothing beyond the superficial. Hopefully your scar healed well, but we need to look beyond the superficial surface scar and whether there was breakdown of the wound or infection. It goes deeper than that. The incision for a caesarean section cuts through seven layers of tissue, including skin, fat and fascia and, of course, your uterus. If you are so inclined (I am!) you can watch jaunty little videos online where people replicate this with playdoh or cake. It's either fascinating or horrifying, depending on your perspective. Either way, it highlights just how deep that scar goes and that surface healing is not the full picture. Sometimes the scar will look nice and neat but you may still suffer pain, mobility or even continence and prolapse issues due to adhesions: tissues 'sticking' together.

Sometimes you can have issues with the surface *as well as* the scar tissue underneath. Hypertrophic scars and keloid scars are formed when your brilliant body is working overtime to heal, creating more tissue than is needed, which will become raised. Keloid scars are made from thicker collagen fibres and tend to 'spill over the sides' of the original scar, while hypertrophic scars stay within the parameter of the first scar. You may be genetically predisposed to keloid scars and they can be difficult to prevent. Multiple studies show that the darker your skin colour, the more likely you are to have keloid scars. Most of the studies I looked at were undertaken in the US, and all report similar findings: *'Compared with whites, keloids were significantly more common in African Americans and in Asians'.*[23] This particular study also highlighted that uterine adhesions were more likely with keloid scars (I'm guessing that what happens with collagen being 'over-zealous' on the surface is mirrored internally), which could mean additional pain and mobility issues for women from black and brown communities. Scars sometimes form quite some time after the original tissue trauma, so try to avoid scratching or further damaging the skin and make sure the scar is fully healed before attempting any scar manipulation.

C-section scars can also cause endometriosis, but this is very rare (around 0.03-1.08%[24] of women who have had caesareans or other gynae surgery). When endometriosis results from a caesarean scar, the medical name is *incisional endometriosis*. Endometrial tissue can build up along the scar, leading to painful adhesions that can occasionally have an impact on fertility or make periods more painful. Endometriosis should not be confused with the very similar sounding 'endometritis', which is infection of the inner lining of the womb, and is more common with caesarean sections.[25]

Of course, scar tissue forms with any scar, not just a caesarean scar, which means that even though you may (hopefully!) not notice (or even look for, as most of us don't tend to have a gander at our nether regions very often, if at all*) any scar on your perineum – there will still be scar tissue underneath the superficial scar. Luckily there is scant evidence about keloid or hypertrophic scars in this area, which I am hoping means they are incredibly rare and this is likely because the skin and tissue of your perineum is very different from the skin on your stomach. However, something called 'granulated tissue' can form. This tissue is red and sore and may bleed and, again, is caused by the body over-compensating to help you heal. Your body is truly marvellous but maybe needs to be a little less over-zealous with its collagen! This tissue should heal on its own, but if you continue to feel very sore near the episiotomy/tear scar and there is a raised red area then you will need to get checked out again and may need something called silver nitrate applied to the granulated tissue, which will (painlessly) break it down. Very rarely, it may need to be surgically removed. Other scar tissue from a perineal tear or episiotomy can also form adhesions to other layers of underlying tissue, which can lead to discomfort, including painful sex.

---

* Midwife Sophie Hiscock does recommend getting a mirror and having a look. She is confident that it won't be as bad as you think. As she says, 'a gnome hasn't grown down there!'

## MUM BUM

I remember seeing a photo, about one year after the birth of my first son, of me carrying him in a sling on my back. He's asleep, we're on a coastal path and it's beautiful. I texted my friend who sent me the photo 'Great pic – but where is my arse?!' It had disappeared, leaving just a baggy expanse of unfilled denim in its wake. So, where did it go? Well, like most women my posture changed with pregnancy, and not for the better. A heavy frontage can tilt your pelvis forward, making you tuck your bum underneath, which can make hip flexors at the front overactive and tight and the glutes under-active, leading to poor muscle tone and weaker pelvic floor muscles. While you may regain some of your natural curvature after the baby is born, carrying and nursing your toddler – and general slumping because you are so knackered – can further weaken this area. Fat distribution of weight gained over pregnancy varies from person to person but, if you now have a flat butt, it might be that the Gods of Trunk Junk did not favour you and instead concentrated on distributing fat elsewhere, which can also give the impression of a more deflated peach. Also, the fat stores you built up in pregnancy will deplete (potentially more so with breastfeeding and exercise). According to obstetrician Clive Spence-Jones, the make-up of this fat is also different and is affected by oestrogen levels in pregnancy, making it 'softer' or less firm. Because of the natural effects of ageing on skin and muscle, this may all be more noticeable if, like me, you come to pregnancy later in life. While researching this, I stumbled – rather horrified – on an article which presented pictures of famous women's derrieres *before* and *after* having a baby and trying to show (not always massively convincingly) that the 'after-bum' was flatter and less attractive. I must admit, it did tickle me a bit to think of the poor sod who had to trawl through red carpet photos looking for evidence of a flatter backside. What an assignment! That said, the standards women are held to are ridiculous and this article was peak tabloid twattery. Also, I'm as vain as the next person, but if a slightly flatter arse is the worst of your problems? I'd say you're in luck! However, maintaining strength in your glutes is really important to keep your body working optimally, so a well-executed squat routine is not out of the question. I started doing mine again after seeing *that* photo, so I'd be a hypocrite if I said 'just love the skin you're in!'. I mean, I want you to do *that*, but I also know the reality of wanting that skin (and fat and muscle) to be doing their best to prop you up… oh okay – and to fill out your 501s.

## MUSCULOSKELETAL ISSUES

To be honest, I wasn't sure what to call this section. I spoke to a friend, Gemma Dawson, who wears three professional hats as an osteopath, a Pilates instructor and a 'Mummy MOT' (pelvic health) practitioner, who has also helped me campaign for better postnatal care. I had so many questions that spanned top-to-toe, that it became a 'general body' chat rather than the 'musculoskeletal' focus that I originally envisaged. As Gemma says, 'everything is connected'. Our bones, muscles and fascia (a thin casing of connective tissue that surrounds and holds every organ, blood vessel, bone, nerve fibre and muscle in place) do not work in isolation. You may have heard the term 'referred pain' before, which helps explain this. Trauma, tension and weakness in one part of the body can adversely affect another, seemingly unconnected, part of the body. As Dr Aviva Romm (also a midwife and a herbalist) says, 'It's so easy to get the nursing-mom shoulder, holding-the-baby shoulder, sleeping in funny positions if you co-sleep – all of that stuff affects your posture, and that can start to make you hold more tension in your body'.

## OUCH

Unfortunately, pain can sometimes continue for a lot longer than the first weeks or months. This can be because of a difficult labour, postural issues, the rigours of new motherhood, stress and tension, hormones still being out of balance or, more likely, a combination of these things.

As well as carpal tunnel, neck and shoulder pain, you may get the 'ouchies' in the lower regions of your back, pelvis, hips, legs and feet. So, everywhere, then? Um, yes. *Sometimes*, for *some* people. Remember just as every birth is unique, so is every postpartum healing journey. Below are *some* explanations for a few of the more common 'ouchies'.

*Coccydynia.* This one is close to my heart. Not literally, obviously. My anatomy knowledge is not that bad. Coccydynia is pain in and around your coccyx or 'tail bone'. I had this pretty severely after sustaining a hairline fracture of my coccyx when snowboarding. I can remember walking from the slope to 'the X-ray man' in the snowy Alpine village where I was living and working. I say walking, but it was more like a stooped shuffle. I dropped my keks and had an X-ray and he told me rather impassively that I had a hairline fracture and then waved me away. Quite clearly he saw this all the time. I was in agony. It was made worse when, during some 'seasonaire' high jinks, later in the season, a rather rambunctious night out culminated with me being dropped from a great height on to the corner of a table. My poor, broken-ish tailbone took the brunt of it. This was almost 20 years ago, and it's only in the last few years that I've stopped feeling reminders of that pain. So, if you are suffering with this – I have quite literally felt your pain!

Coccydynia can be caused by postural changes in pregnancy, such as the tucking of the tailbone that can happen, as well as pelvic floor issues, such as tightness. It can also be caused by trauma during childbirth, such as bruising, dislocation and, very occasionally, fracturing. Sitting upright breastfeeding with this injury can be really uncomfortable, so it may be necessary to practise side-lying feeding to relieve the pressure. You can also take painkillers (discuss with your healthcare provider) and use a 'doughnut' cushion to sit on. Icing the area may also help relieve some of the pain. Fortunately, time and rest will help the coccydynia heal in most instances. If the pain continues, you could consider seeing a chiropractor or having steroid injections.

*Sciatica.* Compression of the sciatic nerve is often caused by issues with the spine such as a herniated (slipped) disc or spinal stenosis (a narrowing of the spaces within your spine). Sometimes you already have this issue, and sometimes pregnancy and childbirth can bring it on. Often characterised as a burning or shooting pain that radiates from your lower back into your buttocks, legs and feet, it is often felt on one side of the body and you can also experience numbness and tingling in the affected area. Moving, bending, sneezing and coughing can all make this pain worse. Weak back and stomach muscles, coupled with long periods of being sedentary, can exacerbate back problems, including sciatica.

*Piriformis syndrome.* According to spineuniverse.com, piriformis syndrome is often mistaken for sciatica, but although the effects are very similar their cause is different. The piriformis muscle is a pear-shaped muscle in the buttocks that reaches from the base of the spine to the top of the thigh. If this muscle is tight it can compress the sciatic nerve and this pain can radiate all the way down the leg. This muscle tightness in the postpartum period is due to changes during pregnancy which both shorten and put pressure on the muscle. A 2013 study concluded that 'Piriformis syndrome should be suspected in any patient with symptoms of hip or sciatic pain, especially after pregnancy'.[26] Which leads me to...

*Pelvic pain.* I was on a pre-baby getaway before baby no.1, at about 30 weeks pregnant, when I turned to my husband over a romantic candle-lit dinner, and said 'I feel like I've been punched in the fanny'. I had no idea what it was and Dr Google diagnosed me with all sorts of utterly terrible potential disorders. A trip to the GP on my return enlightened me: it was, in fact, Pelvic Girdle Pain (PGP), also sometimes referred to as SPD (symphysis pubis dysfunction). As your pelvis softens to enable the baby to grow, it can become more unstable and this can cause you pain. If you have a diastasis (separation) here it can be even more painful. SPD usually 'calms down' after childbirth (if you are yet to have your baby, it is definitely worth letting your healthcare team know that you have SPD as your legs should not be at a wide angle for the birth'), but not always. Sometimes, the pain and instability can be exacerbated by childbirth and can also continue for years afterwards (one – albeit small – study showed the prevalence of ongoing issues to be around 10%[27]). The study is very clear on its strengths and weaknesses, and that more research in this area is needed, but the main take-away was that if women are not 'symptom-free' by six months postpartum, then they probably need 'individualised treatment to prevent long term pain'. This is another reason why it is a good idea to push for a referral to a women's health

---

* On this note, it is absolutely worth checking out Dr Gloria Esegbona and 'The Art of Birth', in which she demonstrates how keeping the knees closer together during birth actually enlarges the pelvic area, making birth easier. It is fascinating and I wish more people were aware of this.

physio. If you start experiencing this pain, keep your knees together as you get in and out of cars, take stairs slowly and try sleeping with a pillow between your knees.

## PELVIS AND VAGINA

Let's face it, there's *a lot* going on down there during and after pregnancy and birth. There are no two ways about it, if you have been pregnant and especially if you had a vaginal birth – you are likely to encounter some issues with your pelvis and/or vagina in the proceeding years. I mean, it stands to reason – you have just housed a human in your pelvis and then pushed it out of your vagina or had abdominal surgery. The very notion that this would not/should not have an impact is unhelpful in itself. This leads women to believe there is something wrong with *them*, rather than this being a common occurrence. Common, however, does not equate to normal. Common means it happens to most women; normal means that the after-effects of this are *fine* and we live our lives without seeking treatment. We are often told that 'these things happen' after having a baby when it comes to pelvic pain, discomfort and incontinence and this is Category A Fobbing Off. We absolutely do not need to resign ourselves to a lifetime of pelvic problems or embarrassment. Nor should we necessarily sign up for a lifetime supply of pads when so many causes of incontinence post-baby can be, effectively, cured.

It is worth noting that some pelvic and continence issues can cause a lot of distress, and this is not yet widely recognised or understood. Many studies show a link between continence issues and depression, and the MASIC Foundation reports that 45% of the women they surveyed said that they experienced depression as the result of a birth injury. If this is you, or someone you know, don't suffer in silence. There are organisations, like MASIC and Make Birth Better, that can help you.

*Appearance.* I'm not sure many women are that familiar with the appearance of their vulva and vagina *before* birth, so why you'd suddenly want to go all Inspector Clouseau (and, let's face it, that probably is the level of expertise we're talking about) directly after you have expelled a human, I do not know. But we know that you do.

And Midwife Sophie thinks that you should anyway. So, what should you expect to see? Well, any bruising or swelling from the birth and stitches should have gone down in the days or weeks postpartum. The opening of your vagina may look a bit wider (or it may not! there is nothing conclusive on this) and you may also be able to see scar tissue on the perineum. You may find that your whole undercarriage is darker than before, as pregnancy can cause long-lasting hyperpigmentation.

Your vagina was built to accommodate childbirth. You have been told that it is 'elastic', but how does that work exactly? Well, your vagina already shapeshifts for sex, becoming longer and wider, and part of the mechanics of this is how the 'vaginal rugae' (accordion-type folds) lengthen. They do the same (but to a larger degree) during childbirth, which means they are also primed to return to form afterwards. The hormones of labour and the uterus contracting enable the smooth muscle fibres in the vagina to disconnect and stretch. This is why fast second stages of labour (although they *sound* brilliant) are not always best for the mother, as it does not give the vaginal tissues enough of a heads up to relax and stretch – which can lead to more pain and tearing. Equally a very long second stage can cause too much stretching. To what extent a vagina 'pings back' depends on many things including genetics, length of labour, size of baby and whether you had an instrumental birth. According to the *Maternal, Fetal and Neonatal Physiology* book I (partly) ingested: 'After a vaginal delivery, the vagina is edematous [abnormally swollen] and relaxed with decreased tone and absence of rugae. The vagina gradually decreases in size and regains tone, although never returning to its prepregnancy state. By 3 to 4 weeks rugae have begun to reappear, and edema and vascularity have decreased. The vaginal epithelium [inner lining] is generally restored by 6 to 10 weeks postpartum.'

Another little nugget I picked up during my research was that although your cervix closes after the birth, it remains a different shape from a woman who has never given birth. The opening becomes a slit shape (sometimes referred to as 'smiling' which I think is a bit lovely) rather than an 'O' shape.

One of my favourite women's health professionals online, Dr Janelle Howell, states 'Expecting your vagina to look and feel the same after delivering a baby is unrealistic. Your vagina figured out how to accommodate the expulsion of a human being. It did this with a bunch of stretching, a little tearing, but it did this without breaking. So now, your body gets to tell that story in a way that can be seen and felt. That doesn't mean settling for a damaged body. It means making peace with a different body.'

*Incontinence.* Incontinence is a huge global problem. If you're thinking it's just you – you couldn't be more wrong. Over 400 million people worldwide are suffering with incontinence, with 10% of women and 6–10% of men suffering with combined urinary and faecal incontinence.[28] Some health professionals who work with people with continence issues seem to think these figures could be conservative, as many people still do not 'present' for diagnosis and treatment. Which means people are suffering silently and alone – thinking it is just them. It isn't. And although it *is* incredibly common, it does not have to be your new normal.

Incontinence can be a very brief side-effect after pregnancy and birth, lasting a matter of days or weeks before rectifying. For a significant proportion of women, issues with controlling their bladder and/or bowels can carry on well in to the first year and beyond. So, what exactly is incontinence? It is defined as any accidental or involuntary loss of urine (wee) from the bladder or faeces (poo) or flatus (wind) from the bowel and can range in severity from a small leak to complete loss of bladder or bowel control.

Incontinence can be caused by pressure on pelvic organs caused by weight gain in pregnancy, as well as by pushing and tearing/episiotomy during birth. You are at increased risk of incontinence if you are overweight, have had a vaginal delivery (especially if it was instrumental), have had a third- or fourth-degree tear, and if you have had a significant number of pregnancies. Caesarean sections are not necessarily protective against incontinence: 'a comparison of women who underwent three caesarean deliveries with women after three vaginal births showed comparable rates of stress urinary incontinence, perhaps because of the cumulative effect of pregnancy itself or denervation injury during caesarean delivery.'[29]

Having accurate statistics for urinary incontinence (UI) and faecal incontinence (FI) after childbirth can be tricky (partly down to a lack of research, the study design and reliance on subjects to self-report). Estimates for long-term continence issues range from 20% UI and 10% FI respectively. However, the largest study I could find, which was on UI and included data from other studies representing over 35,000 women, suggested prevalence was actually 32%.[30] Many health professionals that I have spoken to, and sites I have researched (such as the MASIC Foundation) would suggest these figures are conservative, due to a lack of definitive studies and the widely acknowledged complication of women not coming forward with this type of information, due to embarrassment or, conversely, because they believe it to be 'part and parcel of having a baby'. It is and it isn't. The prevalence is such that we must accept (for now!*) that we will likely experience some degree of 'leaking' at some point in pregnancy and postpartum *but* we don't need to accept that that is how things must stay.

One of the issues that may skew data, particularly when that data is reliant on self-reporting and questionnaires, is not only embarrassment, and being economical with the truth, but also that people don't recognise what is happening to them as a continence issue. When I spoke with Elaine Miller, who as well as being a women's health physio is also a comedian who raises awareness of

---

* I say 'accept this for now' as I feel there is a mountain to climb with regards to creating optimal birth experiences for mothers. 90% of women tear in childbirth. We are conditioned, again, to just accept this as an unalterable fact. I don't believe for one second that if 90% of men tore their scrotum when becoming fathers, that there wouldn't be huge efforts to reduce this number. And don't come at me with 'evolution/big heads/small pelvises' I *know* that, but I also firmly believe that it's not simply down to luck that some women don't tear at all. Fundamentally, I don't believe our 'birthing system' is set up in a way which even tries to maintain bodily integrity for women… #justsayin. *But,* there is work going on to try and reduce the numbers of severe (third- and fourth-degree) tears, such as the 'OASI Bundle' trialled by the Royal College of Obstetricians and Gynaecologists – which has seen a 20% *adjusted* reduction rate. If this is of interest to you, I would highly recommend seeking out the study information on the RCOG website. When I spoke with obstetrician-gynaecologist Dr Sunita Sharma, she was very reassuring, saying that pelvic health is among the identified priorities in NHS maternal care going forward and many changes are afoot.

pelvic health through stand-up comedy, she told me, 'Women go to a pelvic health physio and say they "just leak the normal amount". No amount is normal. Women don't understand that leaking anything is incontinence.'

To help you identify whether you may have a continence issue, the following questions might help:

- Do you rush to use the toilet?
- Do you sometimes leak before you get to the toilet?
- Do you sometimes feel you have not completely emptied your bladder or bowel?
- Do you sometimes leak when you lift something heavy, sneeze, cough or laugh?
- Do you sometimes leak when you run or play sport?
- Do you strain to empty your bowel?
- Do you sometimes soil your underwear?
- Are you unable to control wind?
- Do you wake up twice or more during the night to go to the toilet?
- Do you plan your daily routine around where the nearest toilet is?
- Do you wear pads everyday 'just in case'?

If you answered yes to any of these questions, then you may have a continence (or other bladder/bowel) issue and, the sooner addressed, the more likely you will be able to get help to improve function – which will have a positive knock-on effect on the rest of your life.

As I said earlier, the days, weeks and months after childbirth are the right time to start to re-engage and strengthen your pelvic floor muscles, but it is never too late to start. The first step is listening to your body and acknowledging if there is an issue.

*Pelvic organ prolapse.* I remember where I was the first time I heard this term. I was at a Pilates class and the instructor was adapting moves for those 'with prolapse'. I had no idea what she was talking about and so went home and googled it. I was taken aback to find that something so fundamentally challenging, and so prevalent (studies estimate that 15–48%[31] of mothers have some degree of prolapse, but, again, women's health physios generally suspect larger numbers), was news to me. I really think that things like this and incontinence should be talked about not only antenatally, but much earlier as part of girls' education in pelvic health. We should be armed with the knowledge of how to best equip our bodies to deal with the rigours of pregnancy and birth – and, indeed, any load-bearing or high-impact activity. Athletes and armed services personnel can also fall victim to inadvertently damaging their pelvic floor.

Pelvic organ prolapse is what happens when the internal structures that hold your pelvic organs in place are compromised and one (or all) of those organs slips down out of place. This could be your bladder, uterus, small bowel, rectum, urethra, or even your vagina slipping downwards and out of place. There is a sliding scale of severity – from a grade 1 prolapse which means that there has been a slight drooping or movement of the organ, to a grade 4 which means the organ looks like it is protruding outside the body. Obviously, it is wise to try and address a prolapse in the early stages as you may 'catch it' in time to ensure it doesn't get worse and even, potentially, reverse it. This assumes that you have symptoms, but many prolapse cases can be asymptomatic (meaning you don't feel anything). This is another reason why seeing a pelvic health specialist like a women's health physio or a uro-gynaecologist can be so helpful as they can pick this up when assessing you. Research indicates that urinary incontinence and prolapse are most likely in the white population and can be less likely in black women. It is not clear why this is the case, or even if this *is* the case, or whether the research design is not capturing everyone's data and experience equally. This doesn't mean you should skip a women's health physio check-up if you are a woman of colour though: every body and birth is different and they also treat more than just prolapse.

Symptoms of prolapse include: a feeling of heaviness around your lower abdomen, vagina or rectum, a dragging discomfort inside your vagina; lower back pain; feeling like there's something coming down into your vagina; feeling like you are sitting on a small ball; feeling or seeing a bulge or lump in or coming out of your vagina or rectum; blood or slimy mucus after a bowel movement; discomfort or numbness during sex; urgency or issues with 'voiding' when going to the loo; and incontinence. Pain and discomfort may worsen throughout the day, especially if you are on your feet a lot.

You are at increased risk of prolapse if you had an instrumental birth, had a large baby, had a significant tear, have had a lot of pregnancies/births and have a high BMI.[32] You are also at increased risk of developing a prolapse if you have a chronic cough, and there is also some evidence that having hypermobility[33] (the ability to move joints beyond the normal range of movement) can also increase the risk.

*Dyspareunia (painful sex).* Pain during intercourse. Not fun. And, again, not something we should just put up with. Most women will experience discomfort during intercourse the first time that they have sex after having a baby. This is why you should take your time and not feel rushed into it by any expectations from either your partner or wider societal 'norms'. You are bound to feel a little apprehensive, so taking time to connect with your partner and making sure you really feel ready are important. Doctors will generally advise that tissues should have healed enough by six weeks postpartum to attempt to 'get back in the sack', but it is so individual – some women are ready much sooner and some may take much, much longer. It's not a race.

A 2016 study in Australia showed that 44.7% of women report dyspareunia at three months postpartum, 43.4% at six months, 28.1% at 12 months and 23.4% at 18 months postpartum,[34] which seems broadly in line with other studies. This study also implied that operative procedures (including caesarean or tears and episiotomies that needed stitches) and instrumental delivery were factors that increased the risk of pain. Alongside that, maternal fatigue (show me a new mum who is *not* fatigued!) and spousal abuse were also factors. The latter is more common than we might imagine, unfortunately. In addition to this, many women can experience 'vaginal atrophy' (dryness) after birth, due to falling oestrogen levels, which can make sex uncomfortable. Many women fear 'feeling loose' after childbirth, but with swelling, scar tissue and pelvic floor muscles which can often become 'hypertonic' (too tight) due to trauma and as a reflex after being stretched so much, the opposite is often the case. Topped off with tension in the body caused by apprehension about how sex will feel, this can make sex very uncomfortable – at first. With time, lubrication (if needed) and a gentle approach, sex should start to feel enjoyable and comfortable again. If it doesn't, it would absolutely benefit you to go and see a women's health physio. And remember, sex is not just about intercourse!

*Levator ani injury.* Immediately after the birth, you can tell (or, rather those that are caring for you can tell) if you have sustained a bad external tear. They can even tell if you have sustained an internal tear – such as tearing of the cervix or labia (winces). What is not immediately evident – or sometimes *ever* evident – is whether you have sustained a levator ani injury. The levator ani is a complex muscle which attaches to the pubic bone and forms a large part of your pelvic floor support structure. Its primary purpose is to help support the pelvic organs. A study in 2014[35] found that 21.8% of women who had had a single vaginal birth had some kind of levator ani injury and a further study[36] suggests that a forceps delivery, sustaining a third- or fourth-degree tear and/or having a long second stage of labour can all contribute to levator ani injury. It is also suggested that this type of injury can lead to pelvic issues such as incontinence and prolapse. However, we aren't routinely checked for levator ani injury and it may not always be picked up by a women's health physio either. These injuries may not be recognised until months, or even years, later. Although physio Edel McCann did say this *is* something she routinely checks for. We now know it can occur in 10–35% of women after first delivery.[37] MRI and advanced ultrasound can be used for diagnosis, but a skilled physiotherapist may be able to tell if there is a *suspected* unilateral levator ani 'avulsion' by using palpation (touch) and in consideration with other aspects of a patient's full assessment – for example the presence of weak pelvic floor muscles, prolapse, stretchy lax muscles and possibly an enlarged opening of the vagina/ pelvic floor. Bilateral levator ani defects are more difficult to palpate due to the lack of asymmetry, which is where ultrasound may come in useful. There is ongoing research[38] into this area and early findings suggest that physiotherapy can help the muscle gain strength as well as begin to close any gaps between the muscle and the pubic bone. When I spoke to pelvic health expert Kim Vopni, she told me that trials were ongoing to assess whether platelet-rich plasma therapy (a therapy using injections of a concentration of a patient's own platelets to accelerate the healing of injured tendons, ligaments, muscles and joints) might have a positive effect on restoring levator ani function after this type of injury. While research into women's health can be frustratingly slow and limited, it is heartening to hear about this type of research, and there are massive strides forward happening in the area of pelvic health, so do not lose heart.

*Menstruation.* Ooh, the one you've been waiting for! When will I bleed again? As I write this bit, I haven't had a period for almost a year and a half. I don't hate my monthly 'moon times' (it's what I call it with my son) but I also don't miss them! But I know I don't have long before they make a reappearance. I distinctly remember getting my period after my first son, as I was in a car park with my husband faffing about with our one-year-old and I just said, quite calmly I believe, 'I need to get to a toilet, I am literally pissing blood'. Classy. But, alas, I did find my periods were heavier initially. This is not always the case, however, they may be lighter! You may find your periods resume quickly and are broadly the same as before, but many women do experience changes to their usual cycle.[39] If you are not breastfeeding then your periods will likely resume sooner – sometimes just as the lochia ends after around six weeks (occasionally, they may even start before this). If you are breastfeeding then your periods may not return until you finish breastfeeding, or breastfeeds are significantly reduced. This does not mean you cannot get pregnant. Prolactin affects the ovulation process, but you can still ovulate while breastfeeding so do not rely on it as your only birth control! Your periods may regulate quickly, but for others it takes a while and may be linked to age, whether you're lactating and hormone levels.

With the new demands of motherhood, you may find that the run-up to your period is even more draining and, in rare instances, if your mood is very low and you are experiencing other difficult symptoms in the 'pre-menstrual' phase it could be a sign of Premenstrual Dysphoric Disorder (PMDD). PMDD is not common, occurring in around 2% of women, but it can develop after childbirth even if you have never had it before. More than likely, though, any 'unusual' symptoms pre-menstruation will be as a result of your fluctuating hormones and the changes to your lifestyle. Also, do take note of iron levels, and thyroid function if your periods are not resuming or 'behaving erratically'. Maisie Hill talks candidly in her book *Period Power* about how your cycle can affect your mood, energy levels and ability to parent in the way that you would want to. Hill describes the different phases of your cycle as 'seasons' and explains how you may feel during each of these seasons, and why. Your period, and the pre-menstrual run-up, can make you feel a bit depleted and you may also feel that you are not able to engage your pelvic floor muscles as well as normal at this stage in your cycle. If you are breastfeeding, nursing *may* become more uncomfortable at this time, and there may be a drop in supply pre-menstrually too, according to La Leche League. They recommend supplementing with calcium and magnesium in the run up to your period to help with any supply issues – but do check the dose with your doctor or breastfeeding supporter. Any fussing from your baby should be temporary as they adapt to changes in your breastmilk composition.

*Sex.* <Takes a deep breath> Did you flip straight to this bit? Are you freaking out because sex is different now, in a myriad of ways? You are not alone. Many of us talk about our high jinks and various kinks in our single, carefree days, but that candour goes eerily quiet once you add babies into the mix. From speaking with Sam Evans (a sexual health expert, former nurse and owner of sex toy company, Jo Divine) and Catherine Topham Sly (a relationship counsellor), one thing becomes abundantly clear: *things change* after babies. What things? I hear you cry. And when will they *go back to normal*? Every body, every birth, and every recovery is different – and so are relationships. Like so much in this book, sex in long-term relationships, particularly once you have kids, could take up a shelf or more of book space. I'm trying to be succinct about another huge area of exploration, but, generally, *things improve*. So try not to worry.

But first, what changes? Well, at first you will likely be sore... and tired... and maybe touched out. As well as the physical strain of labour and birth, you now have to learn a whole new role as a parent – and this in itself is a physically demanding role. Catherine Topham Sly told me that in most straight couples, where women still bear the brunt of the child-rearing, this not only leads to tiredness, but also, often, resentment. On top of this, there is often a disconnect in how straight couples initiate sex, with men generally seeking connection through sex, and doing so in a spontaneous way, and women needing connection first (through other types of touch and emotional connection) to feel desire and arousal. Women often joke that their husband stacking the dishwasher unasked is the best form of foreplay, but, as the saying goes, many a true word is said in jest. Recognising the mental load, and the mountain of household jobs that many of us shoulder, makes us feel seen and the value and the strain of your 'new role' (if you are initially the primary caregiver and CEO of the Home) is recognised and appreciated. Catherine told me that women often tell her that they have lost their libido when in actual fact, it is not a physical thing (although persistent libido issues can be investigated) but more often than not, their emotional needs are not being met at a level where they can relax and feel desire and desirable.

So, what about *how it feels*? Well, it might feel different. Or it might not. The first time after the birth is bound to be nerve-wracking but there is *no race*. I think we feel like we have to get that first time after birth out of the way, and sometimes rush it. Your vaginal tissue may be dry for a while after birth, especially if breastfeeding (the oestrogen drop), which can make sex uncomfortable. You may also experience pain or discomfort due to tearing or internal shifts, but if this persists you should absolutely get this checked out. You may also find your breasts leak milk at inopportune moments or your c-section scar becomes uncomfortable with friction. The former is nothing to worry about, and completely natural, but you may want to talk about it beforehand so neither of you gets freaked out. Not all women experience pain or difficulty with sex after birth, so don't let this put you off if you are feeling fine. Marketing consultant Erina Lewis says 'It was nice to get back to it after three weeks. It was lovely to have that connection'. Also, the more you do it, the more stretch that allows in your vagina which can help reduce tension caused by the trauma of childbirth. It should get easier and more comfortable. If, beyond six weeks, and if you've 'tried' several times, there is still pain then ask for a referral to a women's health physio.

## VARICOSE VEINS

My Dad's legs always fascinated me, with their bulgy, colourful, twisted veins snaking their way around his calves and thighs. Unfortunately, this seems to be something he's passed on to me (alongside the 'dodgy tooth' – thanks Dad!). You might have become familiar with varicose veins during pregnancy, thanks to excess pressure on veins caused by weight gain and increased blood volume. Relaxin (that ligament loosener) can also sometimes affect the walls of your veins, making them weaker, which adds to your susceptibility to varicose veins. You will normally find varicose veins on your lower extremities: legs and feet. Do they stick around postpartum? Sometimes, yes, but they should shrink and be less bothersome once you lose any excess pregnancy swelling and weight. By three months postpartum, you should see a visible improvement in varicose veins and, hopefully, any achiness or discomfort will have eased. By one year postpartum, your varicose veins may have disappeared. Unfortunately, some are stubborn and do stick around.

## FEET

Your feet often change in pregnancy due to weight gain and the relaxing of ligaments. This can mean feet seem to become 'wider' and sometimes your shoe size will increase. Women expect their feet to return to 'normal' after childbirth, but quite often this is not the case. Your foot arch often drops a certain amount during your first pregnancy,[40] which affects foot/shoe 'size'. The laxity of your ligaments can mean that your foot begins to roll inwards (pronate), which can cause stress on the arch as well. 'Over-pronating' can result in pain throughout your lower limbs. Any swelling you had in your feet and ankles (I looked like I had trotters) should subside pretty quickly after the birth, but your changed gait may have added extra stress on your feet, and may contribute to conditions such as plantar fasciitis (pain in the sole of the foot around the heel and arch).

## CHIMERA

Are you ready for something pretty breathtaking? Research over the last few decades has indicated that long after birth, cells from the foetus (your baby) live on inside you.[41] This phenomenon is called microchimerism, taken from the Greek word 'chimera' (she-goat!) which means an individual made up of cells from more than one organism. Foetal cells have been found in tissue all over a mother's body, including kidneys, heart and thyroid. Dr Amy Boddy studies to what extent the presence of these cells is positive for a mother, and whether it is sometimes detrimental. The current conclusion seems to be that it is a bit of both: a relationship of 'cooperation and conflict'. There are theories that foetal cells help wound-healing in a mother, and may also help promote the production of milk (to be fair, both of these things benefit the offspring, so this would make evolutionary sense). Conversely, it *appears* that higher rates of foetal cells are found in people with autoimmune conditions – which, if I understand this correctly, can be attributed to the foetus being a little overzealous with their cell gifting. Your body does shed a lot of these foetal cells after birth, as your immune system (which has been suppressed to allow the foetus to thrive in the first place) revs back up. However, foetal cells can be found in mothers *decades* after the birth. Equally, maternal cells can be found in offspring at a similar juncture. Maybe store that for info for a retort to a stormy teenager telling you they never want to see you again. 'Never see me again?! Ha! I am literally a part of you.' Where some might get a bit queasy at this potentially permanent physical link, I actually find it quite heart-warming. We are forever connected. What I found particularly beautiful is that studies show that foetal cells that end up in the heart become 'cardiac tissue' – which means they become a part of your beating heart. For anyone who has lost a baby, this could provide a source of comfort. I know it does for me.

# CHAPTER 6

# HOW TO MAXIMISE YOUR RECOVERY IN THE FIRST YEAR

There's a lot going on in your life in the first year after birth. Adapting to being a new family unit isn't easy. Fitting in time for yourself in between the needs of a young baby, other siblings, your partner (if you have one), work, extended family, and so on, can be difficult. But it is necessary. Women are conditioned to put themselves last and much is made of mothers who sacrifice all for their children. Please remember, in the maelstrom of the first year, that you are a person with needs as well. Find any way you can to carve out chunks of time to nurture yourself. If being a mother is everything to you (and believe me, I understand this), I promise that filling your cup before you pour will help make you an even better mother. If you're at the other end of the scale, where the enormity of what you've been through and what lies ahead threatens to engulf you, taking time for yourself is not a 'nice-to-have' – it's critical. If you are struggling with the huge identity shift, the bodily transformation and the new weight of responsibility – taking time to heal and recover will help restore you to feeling more like yourself.

I am aware that I am adding to your 'to-do' list. There were times when I thought I'd scream if I saw another message or ad telling a new mum (me) to prioritise her 'self-care'. Sometimes it just seemed like another thing to fail at. What I would *love* to see is the postpartum environment and early years of parenting being enveloped in such a strong support structure, that self-care (which in some posts, or in some lives – mine included! – can just mean having a proper shower) is just part and parcel of life and you have the space and time to enact it. 'Shouting Self-Care at people who need Community Care is how we fail people' is a phrase, penned by Nakita Valerio, a Canadian academic, writer and community organiser, that went viral on the internet in the aftermath of the 2019 New Zealand terrorist attack on a mosque. While this was in specific response to how the Muslim community may have felt in the wake of the attack, it resonated far and wide – with many marginalised communities. And with new mothers. I heartily recommend seeking out Nakita online to hear about her work. This sentiment jumped out of the screen at me when I saw it. Self-care is so necessary for our wellbeing, but it can also feel impossible to enact. This is where the 'village' comes in. But, in our modern society, we have lost touch with this notion and women are now carrying more and more of the load, without support, and without time for themselves. I hope you have a brilliant network of support already, but if help is not forthcoming then I must gently, and reluctantly, add my voice to the fray. You are important. Your health, your hygiene, your sleep, your sanity, your ambitions and hopes for the future are all important. Your body is important.

## RESIST THE SUPER WOMAN TRAP

Whether you are working inside or outside the home, you are a full-time mum. And this comes with all sorts of time constraints and sacrifices (amid the joy!). It can be very tempting to tend to all of your never-ending chores and the demands on you, feel guilty about 'never quite being enough or doing enough' for anyone, and find yourself truly and utterly depleted. No woman is an island and you may have to make peace with cutting corners, delegating or (SHOCK HORROR) reaching out and asking for help, in order to enable a full recovery from pregnancy and birth and establish long-term good health. Media images of slim, neat, serene, happy mothers with clean, neat, compliant children make it all look *so do-able*. Well, maybe some days it is (for me, maybe one day out of 365 would look like this!) but most of the time, parenting is messy and topknots rule. Make peace with not being perfect, as perfect parents don't exist. This will enable you to eke out a little time and space to prioritise your health – *as well as* theirs.

Getting the balance right between your needs and your baby/ family can be really tricky. It can feel really hard when you are navigating new parenthood and you are not yet sure which parenting style best fits you. We live in a culture where 'routines' are still regularly advocated as the best practice model of parenting. And I can see why that happens: 'responsive' or 'attachment' parenting can be really hard and exhausting when we don't live in communities which adequately support us. That said, for me personally and for midwife Sophie Hiscock, going with our instincts rather than against them and practising responsive breastfeeding and (safe) co-sleeping was key to our emotional wellbeing and enabling us to get enough sleep to function. However, I am very much 'each to their own' – without the village support structure we desperately need, you have to find a way through that works for your family.

I read another really good quote online, by Becky Vieira, which summed it up for me: 'Society started referring to moms as superheroes because it was easier to sit back and let us do everything while making it seem like a compliment rather than taking things off our plates, or actually stepping up and helping us'.

All that said, there are some things you can keep an eye on that will help you keep the whole show on the road however you are parenting.

## HYDRATION

It's boring. It's simple. It's small.

I almost never drink enough water, so I am a massive hypocrite. But, if you do *one* thing – do this. It affects everything. Your ability to heal. Your energy. Your skin. Your digestion. Your pelvic health. Your ability to focus. All of this is improved with adequate hydration. I keep thinking of ways to up my fluid intake. Things like lovely herbal teas or lovely new bottles. They work for a while and then I fall back into bad habits of racing around like a blue-arsed fly, making sure everyone else has what they need, and not delivering on the *one* thing my body needs for survival. Why is it so hard to fulfil this one teeny tiny, crucial task? I don't know but I will keep trying, as it is one piece of advice that I feel 100% confident in doling out. It's free, there are no side-effects, absolutely everybody needs it, it is a freakin' life *elixir* and did I mention it's free? So, in order to practice what I preach I hereby commit to:

- **Buy a new kettle** (I hate drinking cold water, so teas or plain hot water – thanks Hannah! – are the only way)
- **Buy a water filter** (I live in the south-east and the tap water is rank)
- **Place lovely sports-style bottles** about the house daily and then actually drink the water and then *wash the bottle* – rinse and repeat.

It can't be that hard – right?

## GO AND SEE YOUR GP

If your postnatal check was a blur, or you forgot to go, or you were fobbed off – it may be an idea to try again once you have (hopefully) had a little more sleep and can perhaps leave the baby with a trusted family member or friend. If you are suffering from any lingering issues, from continence to pain, from low mood and anxiety to flashbacks, or if you're struggling to lose weight, struggling to sleep, or just struggling in general – now might be a good time to speak to your GP. They are there to help you get back to health. I cannot stress enough that if you go to your GP and feel unheard, misunderstood or dismissed – try another. And keep trying until someone hears you. I know this can be exhausting and frustrating but, unfortunately, research shows that women's pain is often minimised and misunderstood. My friend Claire kept persevering throughout her first couple of years postnatal, knowing something wasn't right with her recovery. Her energy levels were shot, her milk never came in and her periods only briefly returned. Eventually, after being misdiagnosed with a thyroid issue, Claire found a private endocrinologist who confirmed her hunch that it was Sheehan's syndrome. This is said to be incredibly rare, and is caused by excess blood loss or extremely low blood pressure during/after labour, which affects the pituitary gland. Symptoms often mimic thyroid issues. Claire refused to believe it was a thyroid issue, as she kept being told, and she kept going until she got answers, and the treatment, that she needs.

When I spoke to GP Dr Eloise Elphinstone, she advised that it is fine to seek out another GP at your practice if you are not feeling understood by your own GP. You can ask the reception staff or practice manager whether there is anyone with a particular interest in women's health, or perinatal health more specifically. Candidly, Dr Elphinstone also told me that she feels better able to support mothers after becoming a mother herself. Although she had a real interest in women's health before, she can now 'see it from the other side' and she feels that this can sometimes be beneficial too. Another GP check within your first year can also be a good opportunity to talk to your doctor about any complications in pregnancy which may affect your long-term health, so if you had gestational diabetes and/or pre-eclampsia, you could ask if there is a care pathway whereby you are tested annually to check your blood sugar and/or blood pressure, as you are at increased risk. Dr Elphinstone is keen that patients feel empowered to manage their health, and to take some responsibility for ensuring these checks are scheduled.

## ...AND YOUR DENTIST AND YOUR OPTOMETRIST

Dental hygienist Lottie Manahan recommends that you do not put off going to see your dentist and dental hygienist (particularly as you are entitled to free dental care from a dentist for the first 12 months after your baby arrives!) as 'Your mouth is a portal to your whole body. Look how close your mouth is to your brain and your heart. A clean mouth is a must for good overall health. If your body is working overtime on bacteria in your mouth, and all of the inflammation, it is not as capable of fighting infection elsewhere.' Good oral health (including flossing) is also central to long-term health as it can help prevent cardiovascular (heart) disease and even pneumonia (source: Mayo Clinic). I am well aware that finding the time to floss can feel like a chore (especially when you're knackered before bed), so don't let 'perfect' be the enemy of 'good'; have your floss right there in front of you and just do it as often as you are able. Do your standing on one leg balance exercise, or your pelvic floor exercises, while you brush your teeth – and then you are killing two birds with one stone. A dentist will not be able to correct any tooth movement, but they can potentially suggest an orthodontist, or you can refer yourself. Your dentist *will* help you protect yourself from losing teeth, which studies show is more prevalent after childbirth, and help you make changes so that your oral hygiene has a positive knock-on effect on your general health, as well as giving you a killer smile. Calcium is well-known for improving bone and tooth health, but calcium needs vitamin D to be properly absorbed, so do try to ensure you are supplementing and getting some sunshine on your tired bones.

Equally, after the fourth trimester, when hormones should be stabilising somewhat, do go and see your optometrist to check if you need a new prescription and check in on your overall eye health. Your eyesight *may* be affected for a while longer if you are breastfeeding, so it will be worth mentioning this to your optometrist, along with any pregnancy complications like pre-eclampsia or gestational diabetes. Floaters don't generally go away, but they should become smaller and less bothersome.

## ADDRESS ANY BLADDER OR BOWEL ISSUES NOW

Don't put it off. Don't hope it will just go away. As with almost all health issues, the sooner you address a problem and make changes or receive treatment – the better your long-term outcome will be. You don't have to live with annoying problems and you owe it to your future self to at least get checked out.

The best initial course of action is to contact your GP for a chat. If they are worth their salt, they will refer you to one of the following: a bladder and bowel nurse practitioner, a women's health physio, a urogynaecologist and/or a colorectal surgeon. If you can afford to go private, it may speed things up and there are lots of women's health physios with expertise in this area who can help. In the meantime, you can keep a bladder or bowel diary, such as those available on the NHS Squeezy app or via the Bladder and Bowel Community – also, try to make changes to your diet (see p42) to help with better bladder and bowel function. You can also access something called a 'Just Can't Wait' card (either digital for your phone, or something akin to a credit card). This alerts shop and restaurant owners, or a very long queue at a train station, that you have a condition which means you need to access a toilet more quickly. Other things that can help in the short term are finding a community online, or in person, to discuss your problems and help to find solutions. In my research, I have come across many women online (mostly on Instagram) who are very open about sharing their continence challenges. One such woman is the gorgeous Tor Palfrey, who has experienced multiple prolapse and incontinence issues, and talks about the emotional highs and lows, as well as practical considerations. I am in awe of Tor's refreshingly open, vulnerable and yet optimistic outlook. You can find her online or on Instagram, under the title 'Prolapse, Parenthood and Prosecco'.

### Seek a referral to a women's health physio

When you see your GP, you can request a referral to a women's health physio if you are experiencing issues with pain, discomfort or leaking. Women's health physiotherapists, or pelvic physiotherapists, are trained specifically in assessing and diagnosing pelvic floor and related issues. It is important to see a women's physio whether you have had an abdominal birth or a vaginal birth, as pregnancy itself can affect your pelvic floor and core, and caesarean scars will almost always benefit from some form of scar release or manipulation. A women's physio will run through your pregnancy and birth and go over your medical history. She will likely assess you, which involves her (gently!) inserting fingers into your vagina and feeling for any areas of tension, as well as assessing how strong your pelvic floor is and whether you are correctly doing your pelvic floor exercises. It is said that some women do not perform their pelvic floor exercises (sometimes called Kegels) correctly – with many bearing down instead of lifting up, holding their breath or clenching their bottom muscles and also not giving as much attention to releasing their pelvic floor. These assertions are often made by women's health physios, who are taught to assess pelvic floor strength and functionality. However, a 2013 study[42] suggests most women *do* perform these exercises correctly, especially when given a verbal cue. Either way, it is good to get reassurance on whether you are doing it right or not.

When I spoke with Edel McCann about the women she sees in clinic, it became clear that tension in the pelvic floor can cause just as many problems as muscles that are stretched and/or too weak. We often think of a postnatal body as soft, weak and wobbly, with a belly that was pulled taut around a baby now more of a jiggly mass. This is a bit of a misconception though, as trauma from birth – whether that be scar tissue or tension from psychological or other physical trauma – can cause tightness not only in the pelvic floor, but also throughout the body. In addition to this, you may be frantically working your pelvic floor in an effort to strengthen the muscles while actually making these muscles too short and taut. You may think that constantly 'holding' your pelvic floor up would help strengthen the muscle, but actually overworking the muscle can cause it to weaken and not perform properly when you need it to. Imagine doing a bicep curl and just leaving it there... beyond it looking all kinds of weird, and being deeply inconvenient, that muscle would get soooo tired. Hypertonic (tight) pelvic floor muscles can lead to all sorts of pelvic issues including hip and back pain and incontinence. One woman that Edel treated was experiencing moderately severe issues including stress urinary incontinence and urge incontinence, which resulted in her leaking urine during orgasm. She also had a mild bladder prolapse and all of this was impacting her quality of life and ability to exercise. These issues had been going on for almost a year post-birth before she sought private physiotherapy. When she was seen by Edel she had been prescribed medication for an overactive bladder by her GP and had been to several healthcare practitioners who had told her to do her Kegels religiously. She had become a bit obsessed and was so diligent with it that, after being assessed by Edel and being told to rein it in on the Kegels, she felt really apprehensive about stopping. Edel prescribed more relaxation-based 'down training' techniques that would help release tension in the pelvic floor, including breathing and specific stretches. After three months of this type of training, the woman's prolapse symptoms improved greatly, she was able to run, and most importantly, the urinary leaking, both stress and urge, had stopped. She also no longer required medication. Edel advised that she could gradually reintroduce pelvic floor exercises back into her routine, to maintain strength, but with more focus on the release and 'letting go' element, to reduce any pelvic floor tension going forward.

If you are experiencing real difficulties with prolapse and/or incontinence, your women's health physio might suggest a pessary. There are several different types of pessary (silicone, latex, vinyl) and they come in different shapes, such as rings or cubes. They are devices that are inserted into the vagina to help support pelvic organs. Some women's health physios can fit these, but more often it would be a gynaecologist, specialist nurse or GP. You can also learn to fit and remove them yourself. Some women wear them all the time, whereas others only wear them for high-impact support. As Jane Simpson says in her book, *The Pelvic Floor Bible* 'Vaginal pessaries should be viewed much like a sports bra; you wouldn't dream of going running without your breasts supported, so why not give your vagina the same treatment?'.

### Look after your pelvic floor yourself

I know there will be women reading who will never feel comfortable going to see someone about their nether regions/continence. That's okay! But do find other ways to ensure you are looking after your pelvic floor, whether that be by doing trigger-point release yourself, either with a 'wand' (Thera wand is often recommended) or by following YouTube or Instagram tutorials, like those from Dr Brianne Grogan, or using information from this book, and elsewhere, on how to correctly lift and then release your muscles. Other brilliant books on the subject include *Baby Bod* by Marianne Ryan and *The Pelvic Floor Bible* by Jane Simpson.

Your pelvic floor exercises haven't changed from Chapter 1! *But…* if you're like me, and get a bit bored of doing the same thing, you might want to change your 'cues' a little to keep you motivated. Cues are what you think about to help you locate and engage the right muscles.

Some common 'cues' include:

- Drawing your 'sit bones' together and lifting them up
- Picking up a blueberry with your front or back passage and sucking it up inside you
- Imagine your vagina is sucking up pink milkshake – right the way up your body
- Imagine there is a lift going up inside you (using either your front or back passage) as you exhale and count to 10
- Don't forget to release! Kim Vopni, The Vagina Coach, uses this cue for release: let your bottom bloom (do this on the inhale but do not push down at all).

I also know that very few of us will manage the gold standard of 3 x 20 pelvic floor exercises a day, every single day. I am literally writing a book about it and I almost never manage it – although I aspire to! In the spirit of 'good enough parenting' – there should also be 'good enough self-care'. What we don't need is another stick to beat ourselves with. So, if you manage one set of reps today and do two tomorrow – you're still doing it. If you forget, are snowed under, or are sick, and the days turn into weeks and you haven't done any – don't throw in the towel, start again. These exercises are for life. They should be taught at school-age and become part of our routine like brushing our teeth, but in the meantime (or until the pelvic revolution occurs), just do your best. Good enough is good enough. The Squeezy app is a good tool to help you with reminders. My other tip would be to follow Elaine Miller (@gussetgrippers) on social media, if you use it, as she is making it her life's mission to remind women to do their pelvic floor exercises. There have been a few times now when I've been mindlessly scrolling and a tweet from Elaine has reminded me to lift and squeeze.

If you feel you may need a helping hand with these exercises, or if you are particularly keen on monitoring your progress, then you might benefit from a device. Pelvic floor trainers are inserted into the vagina, like a tampon, and some not only monitor your strength, but also alert you if you are doing the exercises incorrectly. Some link to an app to provide bio-feedback (literally just feedback on what is going on for you physiologically, in real time) on your progress, which can be hugely motivating. A best-selling pelvic floor exercise device, and one that consistently seems to elicit positive reviews, is the Elvie. You can even get ones that provide electrotherapy to stimulate the muscles. Electrical stimulation is sometimes used by pelvic health physios, especially for women with very weak pelvic floor muscles, and from what I have read it can be extremely beneficial. This type of intervention is commonplace in France, where every postpartum woman is eligible for 'perineal re-education' (a 12-week programme of physio for your abdomen and vagina), paid for by the state. Imagine that? Your healing being made a priority... *incroyable.*

A final word on pelvic floor exercises: *they improve orgasms.* *
Part of me is now thinking, should I have bothered with the hours of research, interviewing and writing and just written this instead?

---

* There's no actual evidence of this, but it is so widely espoused within the pelvic health community that it must be true. Here's hoping!

### Learn 'The Knack'

If you do nothing else for your pelvic floor (although God knows I've tried to convert you!), at least learn 'The Knack'. This is a term a lot of women's health practitioners use. The knack is when you activate your pelvic floor muscles in advance of sneezing or coughing. This happens automatically when your pelvic floor is in rude health, but a compromised pelvic floor (such as after childbirth) can find it difficult to perform this action. The contraction (lift) will help keep you continent during these bodily functions, which exert significant internal pressure. As Stephanie A. Prendergast and Elizabeth H. Rummer say in *Pelvic Pain Explained*, 'You need to contract those muscles right before that increase in intra-abdominal pressure, if you perform the Knack too soon the muscles may start to fatigue and lose power and if you perform it too late you may not have given those muscles enough time to perform a maximal contraction to meet that increased intra-abdominal pressure as it bears down on your urethra and pelvic floor'. These pelvic physical therapists also recommend that you follow this with some 'diaphragmatic breathing' (deep breaths into the side ribs and belly) to enable the muscles to properly relax after quite an intense contraction. Especially if you've just had a sneezing fit with your newly acquired postpartum allergy…

## ADDRESS SCAR TISSUE

Scar tissue needs to be mobile and flexible to ensure it does not adhere to organs or other tissues. I am not sure anyone told me this when I was in hospital and after speaking with several other women about their scars, it seems that this is not a well-known fact. A 2011 study stated that '*The evidence for the use of scar massage is weak* […] *Although scar massage is anecdotally effective, there is scarce scientific data in the literature to support it.*'[43] This is despite that very same study highlighting that participants reported that 90% of surgical scars improved appearance with massage and 45% reported improvements including pain reduction and range of motion. A further 2020 study[44] reported that 'In general, this meta-analysis shows that physical scar management has a significant positive effect to influence pain, pigmentation, pliability, pruritus [itchiness], surface area, and scar thickness compared with control or no treatment'. This study (which was, in fact, a study of a number of *other studies*) admits that it is not without bias, and it also is not related primarily to surgical (and definitely not caesarean or perineal!) scars. So, is it useful? Well, scar tissue around the body, and from different causes, may indeed react differently but this, coupled with insights from women's health physios and women themselves (me included!) would highlight that it is both worth exploring individually and also a prime area for further research.

So, what does scar massage do? Practitioners assert that mobilising the tissue in and around your scar will help prevent adhesions. Adhesions are when scar tissue 'sticks' to internal organs and other tissues during the healing process. This can cause you issues years or even decades down the line, especially if the scar tissue sticks to your colon or bladder. People often think that a c-section birth can prevent continence issues and sexual dysfunction, but this is not the case, as women do report both of these issues after c-section.[45] I have tried scar release myself, and can attest to its transformational effects. The practitioner who worked on my scar, Tracey Allport, is an occupational and complementary therapist with training in MSTR (McLoughlin Scar Tissue Release). Tracey told me about how this technique not only 'frees' the body from restriction caused by adhesions and 'pulling' within the fascia, but also often produces a release from emotional trauma. Women can often experience negative feelings about their birth experience if they have needed a caesarean. Tracey says, 'The beauty of this procedure is that it gently and respectfully combines the mind-body connection, treating the person as a whole. MSTR has a profound effect emotionally and psychologically. Scars can hold many different feelings for the individual and as the scar normalises, the feelings dissipate, and the negative feelings recede.'

I did not have much emotion bound into my scar as it was a calm, planned abdominal birth, but I did notice significant reduction in the appearance of my scar afterwards – so much so that I can barely see it now. Tracey explained to me that because fascia is interconnected throughout the body, and a large scar like a c-section scar 'interrupts' this, then restriction and pain can be felt in all sorts of places, including hips and even shoulders! I asked Tracey about her most surprising results from the treatment, and she said 'A lady who had no sensation after her surgery experienced a full return of sensation after just two treatments. Another client, who experienced a burning sensation on her lower abdominal area after her first c-section, came for treatment after her second c-section. Although the treatment is currently ongoing, the sensation is now subsiding, her clothes no longer irritate her skin, and she is more accepting of her post birth body'. It's worth noting that some practitioners can also perform MSTR for perineal scars.

Scar tissue release is not currently available on the NHS, and private practitioners can be costly, but there are things you can do yourself.

*Self-massage for scars.* When you start out, you want to be going very slowly and gently. Do not start until your scar has healed (usually after 6–8 weeks). You may start earlier if you wish, but ensure your scar is not open, bleeding, oozing or scabby and be very, very gentle.

Lie down with your hands on your scar. That's it. Just get used to your scar and how it feels to touch it, especially if it stirs up any emotional reaction. Breathe deeply and focus on your scar. If even this feels too much, leave it for today and come back to it another day.

Increase sensation around the scar by using different (clean) materials to gently stroke the skin around the scar. You can use cotton buds, a make-up brush or a towel/flannel. This has been said to 'reactivate nerve endings'. Physiopedia says, 'The use of various textures applied to the affected skin can provide tactile information regarding the precise shape and size dimensions of the contact area, contributing to a more accurate somatosensory representation.' There isn't masses of evidence for this relating to c-sections (well, colour me surprised) but I did it myself and I have no areas of numbness around my scar.

Gently walk your fingers along the skin above and below your scar, and as you get more confident and more comfortable, you can push your fingers a little deeper.

Make circles on the skin above and below the scar. Press down when doing this but only to what feels comfortable.

'Pull' the skin up and down, working away from the scar and also side-to-side. This can feel particularly 'pinchy' at first, so go slowly and stop if it is too uncomfortable.

Roll the skin around the scar, so that you are pinching along it like it's a sausage, and roll the flesh between your fingers.

There are lots of excellent resources online for helping guide you through this type of self-massage, including videos by physio Hannah Johnson (www.hannahjohnsontherapies.com), who is an expert in this area. Another excellent resource is The Institute for Birth Healing website (a truly wonderful organisation, run by pelvic physical therapist Lynn Shulte) at www.instituteforbirthhealing.com.

I don't want to frighten you about having a c-section. I have been, largely, fine after mine. Dionne Cummings, a business-owner from Leeds, told me that after five (yes, you read that correctly! And, no, this is not recommended) caesarean births, she still feels fit and well and, although she has some tenderness around the scar, she doesn't experience much in the way of pain or mobility issues that she would attribute to the c-sections.

*Massage for perineal tears.* While there is increasing information on the need for perineal massage pre-birth (and YAY for this, as it is shown to decrease tearing), there is not so much on post-birth perineal massage. Considering that you will likely have scar tissue 'down there', it'd be nice for your post-birth vagina to get as much TLC as your pre-birth one! I'm going to level with you, I haven't done this myself yet and I have a six-year-old scar on my perineum now. But it's on *the list.*

The following instructions are taken from an excellent NHS resource:[46]

1. Start by massaging externally. With your thumb or fingers, apply firm pressure and work along the scar line, across the scar and over the scar in circles.
2. When you feel ready to, you can begin internal scar massage (you may take a few weeks to build up to this stage).
3. Place your thumb, pad side down to the back wall of your vaginal opening and your index finger on your perineum over the scar.
4. Apply a downward pressure with your thumb on to the back vaginal wall and make firm 'U' shapes as though moving between 4 and 8 on a clock face.

5. Take your time and build on these techniques gradually. Stop if it becomes painful.

As you advance with this, you could use another technique, recommended by the Carolina Pelvic Health Centre, which is called 'scar rolling'. Place your thumb inside the vagina and your index finger on the scar externally and massage the scar in a circular motion between your fingers like you are rubbing a pearl.

People use many different 'solutions' to change/minimise the appearance of their c-section scar. I have not been particularly bothered about mine so have just used a bit of rosehip oil to massage it, but I hear many positive reports about silicone strips. Silicone gel sheets claim to *'induce hydration and regulate collagen production at the scar site to soften and flatten scars'* and if the Amazon reviews are anything to go by, they seem broadly effective. You may also be able to request these from your GP, as they can be useful when dealing with itching skin around the scar. You must ensure that your scar is healed and not open anywhere before you start using it, and ensure that you keep the gel strips clean if you are reusing them. There are other methods of reducing the appearance of scars too, such as laser, skin-needling, ultrasound, injecting steroids and even surgery, but these seem to elicit very mixed responses. As with any kind of procedure or treatment, do your research. However, if you have a keloid scar or a particularly hypertrophic scar, it may be worth asking your GP for a referral to a dermatologist, as scar massage and release might not give you the aesthetic results that you want.

## MINIMISING 'THE SHELF'

Depending on how large and uncomfortable your c-section overhang is (*if* you have one, not everyone does), there may be things that you can do to minimise its appearance. The first action would be to try and ascertain the degree of diastasis recti, as engaging and healing any tummy gap will help overall strength and may change the appearance of the overhang. You can try to reduce belly fat by reducing overall body fat (you cannot target one area of the body for weight loss, although minimising sugar and stress *may* have a direct impact on 'fat around the middle'*). You can massage your scar to ensure that fascial tightness is not causing your belly to protrude more. With regards to exercises, it may be tempting to try to 'crunch' the belly away, but almost everything I have read suggests that this will actually cause more harm than good. As we've said previously, crunches and planks are not inherently bad for women who have given birth, but they do need to be approached carefully, in a timely manner, and ideally with input from a postpartum fitness expert. The MUTU (MUTU stands for 'Mum Tum') system, created by Wendy Powell, is widely recommended, along with Jenny Burrell's Holistic Core Restore, for helping women regain strength and an aesthetic they are more comfortable with after birth. Both of these programmes focus on working the deep abdominal muscles, posture and breath work. Grace Lillywhite, of Centred Mums, is unequivocal that you should always do a core rehabilitation programme before embarking on other exercise after birth. Give yourself time with this one, and ensure you have the basics of breath, posture, rest, good hydration and nutrition in place, as these are the building blocks for fitness.

It can take quite a while for a c-section 'pooch' to reduce, maybe even a couple of years, so be patient. Whole-body conditioning, coupled with release work (so perhaps a mixture of yoga and Pilates) and whatever other exercise you enjoy, will generate the best results. As with many things, surgery *can* be considered, and there are loud whispers about just how many celebrity mums have 'tummy tuck' (abdominoplasty) surgery after pregnancy, particularly if they have had c-section births. Proceed with caution, however: surgery should never be undertaken lightly, even if you can afford it. As well as all of the usual side-effects and complications that any surgery can produce, you may end up making things worse internally by increasing scar tissue. Always do your research on surgeons and ensure they are accredited.

---

* This is a widely acknowledged hypothesis, although studies appear inconclusive.

## MONITOR YOUR MENSTRUAL HEALTH AND BIRTH CONTROL

Menstruation will likely occur within your first year postpartum, and if it does not, you may want to flag this to your GP. You can be fertile as early as three weeks after the birth of your child, even if you are breastfeeding. Your GP will likely have broached contraception with you at your 6–8 week check-up. The reason GPs are so keen to talk about birth control so early on, is partly because some women get caught out and fall pregnant unexpectedly, but also because they are trying to protect your long-term health. Ideally, your body needs a gap between pregnancies to recover, especially if you have any health conditions. Dr Eloise Elphinstone says 'Getting pregnant early after having a baby can be physically and emotionally really hard. Talking about contraception is important, but the most important thing is choice. However, some women aren't ready to talk about it and that's fine, they can talk about it when they are ready'. The *JAMA* medical journal published a paper in 2018[47] which highlighted that 'birth spacing', ideally allowing more than 12 months between pregnancies, can help with both maternal and infant mortality and morbidity. Older papers from the 1980s focused on hunter-gatherer communities where women often breastfed children for three years or more and birth spacing generally fell into this pattern, with 3–4 years between births. However, we don't all have the luxury of time (geriatric mums like me, for example, have to try to crack on!).

If you are not keen on medical birth control, tracking your cycles when they start again can help you have some level of control over falling pregnant. There are many apps that you can download that will help you do this (including some that purport to be as effective as condoms), but you can also just track on your own calendar. As well as monitoring when you are ovulating/fertile, you can also begin to track how your mood and energy levels fluctuate through your cycle, which can have a knock-on effect, not only on your ability to exercise and what you'll want to eat, but also how you are able to parent and/or work. As I've mentioned before, Maisie Hill writes brilliantly about this, and I have also found Lisa Lister's books (*Code Red* and *Love Your Lady Landscape*) really helpful. To distil the main idea around cycle tracking into a digestible chunk for this book is tricky, but essentially, in week one of your cycle (from the first day of bleeding) your oestrogen and progesterone levels will be at their lowest but will start rising, which means you may gradually feel increased energy and focus; in week two – as your body prepares to ovulate (everyone is different regarding timing of ovulation, but somewhere around 14 days after the first day of bleeding) you may get a surge of energy and brighter moods; in week three ovulation leads to a peak in your hormone levels, but they drop quite rapidly after ovulation, which might mean you begin to feel more tired and sluggish, which will continue into week four as they drop further prior to your next period. Maisie Hill refers to these phases as seasons, which I think is really apt. You don't have to change anything about your lifestyle to reflect your cycle if what you are doing currently works for you, but if it doesn't, tracking can bring fascinating insight into when you can really achieve your goals and when you need more rest and nurturing. Some women adapt their work schedules and their exercise schedules (for example swapping high-impact activity for something more gentle like Hatha Yoga during the lead up to their period), but I appreciate that a lot of women can't do this. Just being conscious of how your body and mind are connected at this point might allow you to cut yourself a little more slack, or get an earlier night, for example, when you really need it.

If your cycles are erratic, as many are, look at your lifestyle and see if there are any adaptations you can make to your diet, exercise, sleep and stress, as these factors play into your cycle – it's not always just your hormones regulating. Make sure you are getting enough vitamin B and vitamin D. A good Vitamin B complex supplement will likely help, but you can also get vitamin B from dark green leafy vegetables, meat, shellfish, dairy products and some fortified plant milks.

You can take a test on the NHS website to assess whether your heavy periods are in the range of 'normal', or not. We know that period flow can change postnatally, but a big change can sometimes be the sign of an underlying condition and may need further exploration. If you are experiencing really heavy bleeding (menorrhagia) and cramping postnatally, you may find that using contraceptive hormone treatment, particularly an IUD (intrauterine device, such as a copper coil), can help alleviate symptoms. You can have this fitted from four weeks post-birth and it should not interfere with breastfeeding.

Sometimes, over the counter anti-inflammatories, or even anticoagulants, might be suggested, and can help. None of these come without potential side-effects, however. Sometimes IUDs can actually make your flow heavier. If you are confident there is no underlying condition (such as fibroids, a thyroid issue or polycystic ovaries, for example) and prefer a more natural approach, I would highly recommend looking up Nicole Jardim, who writes and podcasts about 'fixing' your period, from a holistic perspective. Traditional wisdom (and, unusually, an actual clinical trial[48]) point to the use of ginger in reducing heavy blood flow, so this could be worth exploring. Also make sure you are drinking more water and eating iron-rich food (or taking a gentle iron supplement) to help with your energy levels. If you experience fatigue and a foggy feeling throughout the entire month, in conjunction with really heavy periods, then it might be a good idea to get tested for anaemia.

## SEX (AND RELATIONSHIPS)

When I spoke with Catherine Topham Sly (who has written a workbook called *Back in the Sack* about sex after kids), it was clear that rebuilding connection is the precursor for sexual fulfilment after babies. Our relationships change so much with the arrival of a baby, with priorities shifting and both partners often feeling under-supported. Unrealistic expectations can also make things much harder. It might take quite a while for our intimate relations to resume to anything like a pre-kids level, and putting further pressure on both of you won't help. We've established that men often crave sex to feel connected, so it is worth bearing that in mind, as it might help you understand how dynamics change when sex falls down the agenda. If you're both seeking connection, but in different ways, you might be trying to get to the same place with wildly different maps and never meet in the middle. This is not to say that rekindling that spark is easier in same-sex couples. We are all navigating the unknown together. It is worth discussing what makes you feel desire and desirable and building from there. Communication is key.

Feeling desirable is, unfortunately, in our porn-saturated society, very tied up with a 'performance-based' idea of sex, with a woman simply something to be looked at and used as a vessel for a man's pleasure. Catherine said it might be helpful for women, particularly if they are feeling unconfident in their bodies post-birth, to reimagine what sex is for them. Seeing sex as more of a 'mindfulness' exercise, where the focus is on experiencing touch and pleasure and concentrating on the senses – being present in the moment – rather than listening to the noise in your head and wondering what you look and feel like, can help women to begin to enjoy sex again and foster a greater connection with their partner. Remember, sex doesn't need to be serious. It's meant to be bonding and fun. So, if something weird happens, try to have a laugh about it. A loving and understanding partner will want to make you feel comfortable. Also, he (or she) may be terrified of hurting you, so do bear that in mind if you sense any reluctance or trepidation.

Sam Evans advises that we really take our time. 'Wait until you are relaxed and comfortable, ready. There is no rush at six weeks, don't feel pressured by your partner and focus on non-penetrative sex to begin with, kissing, cuddling, intimate massage, masturbation, oral sex. It is important to use an irritant-free lubricant, especially if you are breastfeeding as the drop in oestrogen can cause the tissues of the vulva and vagina to become dry and less well lubricated. Always check the ingredients as many products contain irritating ingredients including glycerin, glycols, parabens, dyes, perfume and alcohol'. Sam recommends using YES organic oil-based lubricant, which she says is ideal for massaging scar tissue and if you aren't using condoms. 'Explore different positions which enable you to control of the depth of penetration. If it feels uncomfortable or painful, always stop and enjoy non-penetrative sex play'. Sam also says that there are sex toys available which can help with things like scarring and decreased sexual sensation. It is absolutely worth finding her online to find out more about this.

Having over-sensitive or leaky breasts might bother you, so do chat about this and any other areas you might want to be 'no-go' areas that you simply don't want touched at the moment. A c-section scar can be very uncomfortable for a number of weeks, so anything rubbing along it will cause irritation, which is not very sexy. As we've mentioned before, the trauma of birth, and scarring, can cause a lot of tension in the pelvic floor and this can take a while to settle down, so things (surprisingly) can feel too tight for sex to be comfortable. At the other end of the scale, if things do feel looser, Sam is keen to point out that you should try and see a pelvic floor physio. Even if your vagina has pinged back (and they do!) to something resembling your fanny of yesteryear, then internally things can have shifted and feel different, so that what felt good before doesn't anymore. Be vocal. Don't endure things that are uncomfortable. If you are feeling unconfident, rather than not 'being in the mood', *tell* your partner. They can't mind-read and remember this is a huge adjustment for them too, and feelings of rejection can surface.

Don't forget that your hormones will be impacted for as long as you are breastfeeding. Some mothers breastfeed for 'extended' periods of time, which may affect not only how they feel about sex, but also how ready they are physiologically. La Leche League Canada states, 'It is not surprising that breastfeeding, which is hormonally driven, would have an impact on sexuality which is also hormonally driven. While the hormones involved in breastfeeding may have a dampening effect on sexual desire in the early months, intimacy is more likely to occur when a mother is feeling rested and supported in her parenting and other roles by her partner'.

Sam also echoes Catherine's advice about communication: 'talk to your partner about how you are feeling about sex so that they can try to understand and allay your fears. They may be worried too. Both of you may be petrified of getting pregnant again, so, if you are in a heterosexual relationship, using a reliable form of contraception is important'. To sum up Sam's advice, I would say: take it slow, talk about things, cuddle, pick comfortable positions and use good lubricants. If all of this is not a recipe for success, and you are experiencing consistent pain, discomfort or more of a psychological barrier, then talk to your GP, as they may be able to refer you for psycho-sexual counselling, consider a prescription for lubrication or some sort of physical therapy/treatment to help you. It is not something you just have to accept. In the meantime, don't stop talking to your partner. Catherine Topham Sly tells me that couples seek therapy on average six years after they would have first benefitted from going. Within that time, more layers of dissatisfaction and ire will have built up that could have been dealt with earlier.

Catherine is aware that couples may be scared about what will come out in therapy, but she says a good therapist will guide you very gently and 'hold you' as you peel back these layers. Equally, she says, once things are out in the open they can be dealt with as 'the unsaid' holds so much power in a relationship. If therapy isn't for you, or is not accessible for you, then Catherine recommends the books *Come as You Are* by Emily Nagoski and *Mating in Captivity* by Esther Perel. Also, if you are considering therapy but can't afford it or access it through a charity like Relate, then some counsellors will offer low-cost options and your local religious centre (yes, really!) might also offer free guidance and advice.

Catherine and I discussed a venture she tried to get off the ground, in which she offered couples antenatal advice about the impact a baby might have on their relationship. She said she was met with stony silence from those yet to have children and effusive 'I wish we'd had this' from those that had. It's funny how we prepare our homes so meticulously for the arrival of the wee ones, but give next to no thought to how to insulate our relationship against such a huge change. I hope Catherine keeps going with that idea, as I think it could have huge benefits.

If you are experiencing issues with intimacy, or your relationship in general, you might find the episode of the Postnatal FAQ podcast with psychologist Julianne Boutaleb very reassuring. She normalises the incredible shift that happens within relationships, both heterosexual and same-sex, when your baby comes along, stating 'It is normal to feel out of sorts with each other. It is normal to lose each other for a while. It will feel negative at times. It is a gift if your partner can see what you need on any given day.' Also, Illiyin (Illy) Morrison, a birth debrief facilitator (@mixing.up.motherhood on Instagram), is very candid about how having a baby impacted her relationship. I love all her posts on this, but this quote is perhaps my favourite, 'Everything felt fragile… I don't think we liked each other too much, the buzz of child-free relationships was gone and replaced with having an annoying flatmate. That was the season. That was the season of my relationship then. I would compare it to the British winter, literally feels never-ending. But Spring eventually comes.'

*Vaginal rejuvenation.* Where to start? What is it? Does it work? Should we bother? Why are we socially conditioned to constantly try and change and improve every little thing about ourselves?

What it is: it can take different forms, but generally it is laser treatment on the vulva and vagina that aims to both plump and shrink tissue and increase moisture. Lasers create small wounds which your body then produces collagen to heal, creating more tautness.

What it isn't: a substitute for a thorough pelvic assessment with a women's health physio, which can address multiple issues.

I was pretty torn (excuse the pun) when I researched this area, as there are real concerns around a treatment that seems to be not well regulated, not thoroughly researched or evidence-based and predicated on women's insecurities. On the other hand, there are so many heartfelt testimonials both online and throughout other media, in which women talk about how laser or ultrasound treatment has 'changed their life'. When I spoke to obstetrician/gynaecologist Dr Sunita Sharma, she said she was absolutely not an advocate for this 'treatment' for postpartum women, as there is no clinical evidence to support such interventions. She says that in the 'acute phase' (immediately after birth) we should be supporting women to optimise wound healing and pelvic floor rehabilitation.

## WHAT YOU WEAR

If you've been wearing a tubigrip, or any other type of postpartum girdle, now might be the time to give it up. They are great for helping you feel more confident and supported, particularly after caesarean sections, but there comes a point when you need your abdominal muscles to start working for you again.

Good footwear is also a must. With arches potentially dropped, pronation (rolling feet inwards) potentially exaggerated and the sheer amount you are on your feet as babies grow up, looking after your feet is important. I know it's boring! Heels are not your friend. You don't need to give them up for good, but try to limit how often you wear them. Decent, supportive trainers that lace up properly are what will really help you. Alternatively, Grace Lillywhite recommends 'barefoot'-style footwear (for walking throughout the day, not for running unless you're already a convert). Barefoot shoes can be expensive, but you can often find cheaper styles on Ebay (not used!).

## EXERCISE

At my leaving do at work before I went on maternity leave the first time, one of my team – a striking and assertive Russian lady who had two children – came up to me and stated quite strongly but in slightly hushed tones 'you know, you *must* go to Pilates after you've had the baby'. I knew she was giving me 'the secret' in some way. I don't think she had offered any other advice or tips on motherhood at all, so this stayed with me. I had dabbled with Pilates and yoga before but, after my first son, I dove head-first into postnatal Pilates and found it a godsend. Not only because it gave me a precious hour to myself (that was *after* I jettisoned the mother-and-baby classes, where I spent most of the hour nursing, cleaning up a poonami, or being crawled over), but also because I began to feel my body shifting back into place. My tired, flat feet were awoken by rolling spiky balls underneath them, my pelvic floor perked up with bridges and careful squats and my back – oh my back! – was released from the stoopy, droopy, achy and concave position it had adopted as I lifted, fed, changed and co-slept. To be honest, I would have paid my tenner just to lie on a foam roller in peace for an hour.

I also ran when I got the chance. I am not a runner but it is free and there is no timetable, so it was something that felt 'do-able'. I do remember my Pilates instructor looking slightly aghast that I was running so soon, but I then found out that she *also* ran, so I felt I had my pass. I have since learnt that there was a period of time when many women's health physios and/or personal trainers did not advise women to run in the postpartum period at all. I now know that it can be associated with increased risk of pelvic organ prolapse and incontinence. Luckily this didn't happen to me, but the thought of it put me right off. Don't despair, runners! There is hope! In the intervening years (in which I experienced recurrent miscarriage and then finally carried to term) health professionals have been working on creating programmes which enable women who have had babies to run again, without fear of damaging their pelvic health. Hurrah! One such practitioner is Emma Brockwell (The Physio Mum), who, as well as organising a women's running club in Oxted, Surrey, has developed a framework, alongside colleagues Tom Goom and Grainne Donnelly, which offers health and fitness professionals some guidelines[49] to help determine when postnatal women can return to running.

When I spoke to physio Edel McCann, she had this advice for women looking to get back pounding the pavements: wait 12 weeks post-birth before attempting a run and make sure you have done the stress tests (listed below) and are experiencing no symptoms (leaking, heaviness) before you go. Running and other high-impact sports are at the top of the pyramid: you need to get the foundations below sorted first, such as strength training. Edel also said 'Find your fence. See what you *can* do without symptoms and then gradually build up and move the fence'. If you are starting from a no-running background, then still do the stress tests below but also start very gently, with something like the NHS Couch to 5k programme.[50]

According to the Return to Run guidance, a postnatal woman should be able to do the following without pain, discomfort (including dragging or a heavy sensation in pelvis/vagina) or incontinence:

- Walking 30 minutes
- Single-leg balance 10 seconds
- Single-leg squat 10 repetitions each side
- Jog on the spot 1 minute
- Forward bounds 10 repetitions
- Hop in place 10 repetitions each leg
- Single-leg 'running man': opposite arm and hip flexion/extension (bent knee) 10 repetitions each side

A pelvic health physiotherapist is best placed to assess you and advise you on the above, and they will also be able to perform additional checks that are outlined in the guidance (such as checking your pelvic floor strength against the Modified Oxford Manual Muscle Testing assessment tool), as running is not advised in some instances if you score lower than Level 3. However, I am well aware that getting the physio sessions you need and deserve is not always easy, so the above is a starting point for those eager to lace up their trainers.

Speaking with Kim Vopni, the Vagina Coach, she suggested that you can up the intensity of your exercise at about six months postpartum, providing that you do not feel any pain or suffer with leaking issues. She also recommended providing your body with a *variety* of exercise. As Jo Sharp said in the context of nutrition, variety is a key factor in health. A variety of exercise will help awaken muscle groups that are feeling a bit left out (weak) and will also reduce the risk of injury as you are not creating too much 'wear and tear' in one place. Beyond that – it *feels good* – and it keeps things interesting to mix it up. As with anything, doing the same thing over and over can leave us unmotivated and stuck in a rut. This struck a chord with me. I get very used to 'fitting in' very specific workouts or exercise 'portions' (mostly revolving around tagging a walk on to the school run or a mini workout in the bathroom before a shower – because I can lock the door and no blighter can get to me!), and I have definitely been stuck in a rut. Kim suggested mixing yoga with doing some gentle weights, but ultimately she was keen to stress that you do *what makes you feel good* and what serves you. It was reassuring to hear Kim say that no exercise was necessarily off-limits. I have definitely been told not to do crunches or planks before, but Kim says it's *the way* that we do them that is important. We generally 'do' crunches in everyday life anyway when moving up and down, especially with small children (even though I still tend to roll to my side to get up off the floor), and so it is best to know how to do them without negatively impacting our body. If at all possible, it would be best to be assessed by a specialist women's pelvic health physio or trainer to ensure you are doing any 'load-bearing' or high-impact activity correctly. This is not always possible for budget reasons, so at the back of the book I suggest some really good instructors to follow online so that you can feel more confident exercising.

During my conversations with Kim Vopni, a couple of things she said really stuck out. The first was about the 'masculinisation' of fitness. We were talking about lifting weights, and she was advocating for light (5–10lb) weights with enough repetitions until you begin to feel tired. She lamented how 'lifting weights' was generally seen as a something men do and that lifting the biggest, heaviest weights was the ultimate goal. The Pelvic Guru, Tracy Sher, also talks about how exercise is 'male-centric', and that some exercise techniques (such as deep inhalation and breath-holding on lifting heavy weight, or posture for squats – see below) can create too much intra-abdominal pressure for women, which puts strain on the pelvic floor and pelvic organs. She also highlights how our bodies change, including flexibility of tissue, during our menstrual cycle, which can cause us to over-stretch. I really liked the idea of feminising my fitness routine to work *with* my body, around my cycles and where I am in my life right now and so I (quite literally) go with the flow and do stronger moves when I have higher energy and more gentle, releasing exercise (or none at all!) when my energy reserves feel depleted.

If you are experiencing conditions which make you feel very tired, make it difficult to weight bear or which make your joints feel achy (like arthralgia), swimming classes (with baby or without) might help you to feel active without straining or exacerbating the issue. Mother and baby classes are often held in warm pools (like hydrotherapy pools), and I did find this to be a lovely bonding experience too. A woman on the Versus Arthritis website extolled the virtues of aquanatal classes, so some form of aqua aerobics (or something gentler) might also be a good shout. If you had pelvic girdle pain (also called SPD) in pregnancy, and are still suffering with it, try to avoid the 'frog legs' motion that goes along with breaststroke. According to SwimTeach.com, 'Swimming with SPD can still be possible by using other strokes or exercises that require minimum leg movement. That's most things that do *not* require a breaststroke leg kick. You can use a float, kickboard or swim noodle to kick using a front crawl or backstroke leg kick, or use the noodle tucked under your arms and just use an arm action without any leg kick at all. The point is, you are getting some movement and exercise whilst avoiding undue pelvic movement.'

It is worth mentioning NEAT here. No, I'm not going to extol the virtues of housework as a workout. Well, maybe a bit. NEAT stands for 'non-exercise activity thermogenesis', which is, essentially, everything that we do that is not sleeping, eating or actual sport. As parents, we do *a lot* of NEAT. Seriously, what woman in her first year of parenting does no exercise at all in a day? At one point in the Covid-19 pandemic, my husband was ill with Covid and we had just moved house. We were all self-isolating in a teeny tiny bungalow, full of unpacked boxes, in the depths of winter, and I did at least 5,000 steps a day. I have no idea how. The recommended minimum step count per day is 10,000, and you can easily rack these up as a parent – by doing the school/nursery run on foot, walking to the park, having kitchen discos with the children and just simple errand-running.

Being sedentary is known to have an adverse impact on your health, but I am well aware how easy it is to get trapped underneath a snoozing baby for hours on end. This is where slings come into their own. Some babies will fall asleep happily in a pram, but mine definitely preferred being snuggled up on my chest and I found walking as they slept helped me with my physical fitness and my mental state. If you build a few hills into your walk – even better! If you are using a sling, again make sure it works for you with regard to comfort levels and that your body can take that load. It might also be worth checking in with your local sling library to trial different slings as some can cause backache. There is usually an experienced 'sling-wearer' there to help show you how to use them. I don't know about you, but finding out about NEAT (and how much energy you expend just going about your daily business!) made me feel sooo much better for not having a strict workout schedule.

Kim Vopni said to me 'People, especially new mums, feel guilty because they don't go to the gym or workout. But you compare a person looking after children all day to those working in an office and then going to the gym for an hour and who is moving more and in more varied ways? Mom life is very busy and movement rich'. So do think about that if you feel you are not getting enough exercise. Chances are you're already halfway there. That said, the joy of having the chance to exercise alone, and to do a form of exercise that you love, should not be underestimated. Many people find running, dancing, boxing or paddle-boarding (insert your favourite sport here… table tennis? Boules?) absolutely critical for their mental health, physical health and overall wellbeing. As part of your postpartum plan, you could talk to your partner, or other support network, about how you will be able to fit in at least one session of your favourite sport a week, once you feel able to.

***Exercise for carpal tunnel and mum thumb.*** Carpal tunnel and mum thumb can both be a real drag. If they are serious, you will hopefully have been seen by a healthcare practitioner and may also be wearing a splint. If not, try the following to help alleviate symptoms:

- Modify how you lift your baby. Mum thumb can be caused partly by repetitive movements, and a prime culprit is how you lift the baby. Instead of lifting by putting your hands underneath their armpits, try scooping them up, with one hand on their back and another under their bottom.
- Modify your breastfeeding position. If you have the full weight of baby's head in your hand, and your wrist is unsupported and at a weird angle, you can exacerbate both carpal tunnel and mum thumb. Ensure you have enough cushions to help take the baby's weight and have hands flat rather than bent at an angle.
- Reducing scrolling and tapping on your phone can help your whole posture, including the already overworked tendons in your wrists and hands.
- Opening and closing fists a few times a day and 'contrast bathing' hands and wrists with ice packs and heat packs may help relieve tension.

***How to squat properly.*** Squats are brilliant for strengthening abdominal muscles, legs, glutes (bum muscles) and also your pelvic floor. However, many of us don't do them properly and so we are not effectively engaging our glutes. For women without prolapse, these should not present any issues. If you do have a prolapse, let your instructor know as they should be able to modify the exercise for you.

For all:
- Everyone is told to stand with feet hip distance apart and with toes pointing forward. However, this is sometimes deemed to be a 'male-centric' stance and, as women's hips and legs are different to mens', it may be more intuitive to have a slightly wider stance with toes rotated out slightly.
- Lift your toes to ensure you can feel what putting the weight 'backward' into you heel feels like. Place toes back down, as splayed as is comfortable.

- Lower yourself down, keeping that feeling of having your weight backward rather than on the front of your foot.
- As you push back up, breath out and focus on pushing your heels into the floor and keeping your shoulders going straight up and down.
- Do 10–15 reps and as you get stronger you could add dumb bells to increase intensity.

For those with prolapse:
- Mini squat: bend forwards from the hip and stick your bottom out.
- Don't go as deep as you would with an ordinary squat.
- Focus on pushing your weight through your heels as you come back up.
- Wall squat: stand with feet approximately hip width apart, your back against a wall and your feet facing forward away from the wall.
- Squat and lower your back down the wall by bending your knees, keeping your knees behind your toes.
- Keep your hips positioned higher than your knees
- You can also try this exercise rolling a Swiss ball up and down the wall behind you.
- Breathe normally, don't hold your breath.
- See Fem Fusion Fitness or Honest Yoga online for more details and videos on prolapse-safe exercising.

*Glute stretch.* If you're working your bum (as above) and if you're not (long periods sitting down), either way it's advisable to give it a stretch. Grace Lillywhite maintains that you can't properly strengthen a tight muscle.

- Lie on your back with your feet on the floor, knees up.
- Place one ankle on the opposite knee.
- Thread your arms through to hold the knee of the leg that is 'up'.
- Gently pull towards you, bringing the other foot off the floor.
- You should feel a stretch in your glute.
- If you pull your leg closer, it will create further intensity.
- Hold for as long as you are able, then release.

*Lazy Angel.* Did someone say lazy? I am in. This exercise is brilliant for new mothers as it takes us out of the 'cocoon stance' in which we hunch forwards around our baby. It helps open up your shoulders and chest and it feels amazing.

- Lie on your side using one arm or a small pillow/yoga block for head support.
- Place your ankles, hips, knees and feet together with your knees bent in front of you at a 45-degree angle.
- Stretch your arms out in front of you with palms together.
- Focus on the out breath, maintaining balance for the spine by gently imagining the belly button sucking inwards.
- Slowly lift your top arm up and over your head, drawing a half circle toward the back of you as your chest opens toward the ceiling. This can feel quite strong so lessen the stretch by bringing your arm closer toward you if you need to.
- Turn your head so that your eyes follow your arm, but keep your knees, feet and hips anchored at all times
- Bring your hand down and round in another half circle until it meets your lower hand again.
- You are creating a circle like movement. Take your time and remember to breathe into your ribs as you move, while maintaining a slight contraction of your abdominal muscles so that your back is supported. If anything feels off, lessen the movement or stop.
- Repeat 8–10 times on both sides, increasing the range of motion, if you can, as you progress.

*Hip action.* Many women suffer with tight hips after pregnancy and, while stretches might work for some, it's really your overall posture that will help alleviate these symptoms. You want to try to not stand with a clenched bum, thrusting your hips forward, but create a more natural curve to your spine with your pelvis in 'neutral'. It can be harder than you think to do this, especially with core weakness and the constant demands of baby wrangling.

If you really need to feel that release, try these super-gentle stretches:

- Lie on a high bed on your back with one leg dangling off – gravity should pull you into the most gentle stretch. Repeat both sides.
- Lie on your front (the *joy* of this, after 10 months of pregnancy!) and bend one leg at the knee. Reach back and hold your foot. Release if it is too intense.

## EAT FOR HEALTH

When I spoke to Jo Sharp, she explained to me that sleep deprivation can affect your ghrelin and leptin (hormone) levels. As ghrelin makes you feel hungry, and leptin makes you feel satiated (I'm simplifying!), having these hormones out of whack can wreak havoc on your eating habits. As we've mentioned before, if you are tired and stressed, you are more likely to reach for quick, sugary snacks rather than a slow-cooked or more nutrient-rich snack or meal. In turn, the quick sugar hit will lead to an energy crash, which will make you feel tired again and possibly even more irritable. It's a vicious circle. I'm not going to be a liar and say I did not get trapped in this cycle. I absolutely did. And I still do sometimes. I got so tired during the first Covid lockdown, with a newborn and a five-year-old at home all day, that I stuffed my face with marshmallows. My husband calls this 'zombie food'. It has no nutritional value. I don't even *like* marshmallows. This feeling of fighting tiredness can last well into the first year and beyond, and can definitely affect your ability to choose healthy foods. It sucks and can feel out of your control but there are little things you can do.

Firstly, to address the fatigue, try opening a window first thing to get light on your face (helps your natural circadian rhythm), take a walk, go to bed an hour earlier, have a bath, or do some yoga nidra. Also, try to give yourself a head start by stocking your fridge with fruit, veg and protein-filled snacks. I don't know if it's because I have kids, and kids are programmed to snack, but I am a snack-monster these days. I try to make sure I have hummus, peanut butter, nuts, apples and dark chocolate to hand in the house as these are my go-to snacks and don't make me feel totally awful.

It can also be really easy to fall in to one of these familiar traps:

- Eating your baby's/children's leftovers. Don't do it. If you're treating that as your main meal, give your body more respect than that –

you deserve better.

- Inhaling your food. Whether it's because you want to eat using both hands and you have a small window of time before baby-bedlam ensues, or you have older kids and they sit still for approximately three minutes at dinner time, we often eat way too quickly. Digestion starts with the mouth and you are not giving your gastro-intestinal tract enough of a heads up if you are gobbling down your food. And we want a happy tummy. Also, your brain doesn't register that you are full for 20 minutes after starting eating. In our household, the plates are scraped and the dishwasher is on by then, which means we regularly over-eat!
- Doing all the cooking. Nothing saps the joy out of cooking like having to do every single meal (which, of course, goes way beyond the actual cooking, as it starts with the meal planning, food shopping, timing and prepping!). It also means we can fall into a rut of having the same meals on rote. Variety is not only the spice of life, it is what helps keep your microbiome happy, and good gut health affects everything. Try to ensure that the responsibility for all meals (*including the planning*) is shared. If you are in a single-parent household, you could consider sharing meals with your parents/siblings or maybe hook up with other families to go over to each other's houses for one evening a week.

The NHS website on healthy eating, 'Eat Well', asserts that 'Most people in the UK eat and drink too many calories, too much saturated fat, sugar and salt, and not enough fruit, vegetables, oily fish or fibre.' So, basically, do the opposite of this to be healthy! Eat good fats (olive oil, nut butter, avocados) rather than saturated fats (cakes, sausages, cheese), up your fruit and vegetable intake, reduce your salt and sugar intake and aim for 2–3 portions of oily fish (or vegan equivalent such as flaxseed/supplement) every week. Oily fish needn't be expensive, like salmon, it could be tinned sardines or mackerel – and if the bones are included all the better, as they're great for calcium.

We talk a lot about cake in those early weeks and months postpartum. I have often sustained myself on coffee and cake (usually coupled with the chance to offload to a friend with a sympathetic ear). I don't want to deprive you of your cake. But I have a hack (of sorts!).

Try a healthy (ish) mug cake. They're cheap, you can make them from whatever you have in, you can add things in to balance your blood sugar (like chopped nuts), and they don't contain additives which are detrimental to your health. My husband thinks they are rank but I love them. I don't use measurements, but here is my go-to mug cake for a low moment:

1.  Half fill mug with flour (I use gluten-free plain flour) and cocoa
2.  Add tablespoon (ish) of oil (olive or coconut) or butter
3.  Add tablespoon and a half (ish) of honey or maple syrup
4.  Add chopped hazelnuts and a piece of dark chocolate
5.  Add a few tablespoons of milk (I use oat) until consistency is sloppy(!)
6.  Microwave for one minute, stir, then give it a further 30 seconds.

The beauty of this is that you can keep trialling and adapting until you find what works for you! You can add banana for more stickiness and potassium.

You can balance this 'indulgence' by making some bone broth. Bone broth is a clear, protein-rich liquid made by simmering meaty joints and carcasses. You can slurp it like soup or use it much as you would stock (in stews, soups and risottos). You can boil and simmer a chicken carcass after a roast or you can ask your local butcher for beef, or other, bones – which he/she may give you for free. Bone broth has been shown to contain essential nutrients which help the body heal and perform optimally, due to its high collagen levels. You can make your broth complicated and fancy, or you can simply cover the bones in the pot with water, bring to the boil, add a bay leaf (I don't really know why I do this, it has some 'cheffy' vibe to it though!) and simmer for the entire day. It can be stored for a few days and even frozen in cubes for 'ready-made' stock.

Here is a bone broth recipe:

-   2–3kg beef bones, chicken carcasses, lamb bones
-   2 handfuls of any onions, leeks, carrots or celery ends
-   1 tbsp black peppercorns
-   A few dried bay leaves

1.  Place the bones and any additional ingredients into a large stainless steel cooking pot, and cover with cold water. The water level should cover the bones sufficiently but also leave a little room at the top of the pan.
2.  Cover and bring to the boil. Reduce the heat and simmer, with lid on. It will take 6 hours or more for chicken and 12ish hours for beef or lamb, although I frequently only leave mine for 8 hours or so and it seems fine. However, the longer you leave the bones to simmer, the more nutrients you get. Skim off any foam that rises to the top. Alternatively, using a slow cooker or pressure cooker can save time and fuel.
3.  Strain the liquid, using a sieve. Use immediately or leave to cool before storing (if you can use glass/ceramic rather than plastic). Bone broth keeps in the fridge for up to a week as a layer of fat will form on the surface and make an air-tight seal.

In his wonderful book, *The Postnatal Depletion Cure*, Dr Oscar Sellerach goes into a lot of detail about how long maternal depletion can last (spoiler: he's encountered women who – 10 years postpartum – he would class as having postnatal depletion), why it happens, and how to try to combat it. Alongside a plea to check for hormone issues and vitamin deficiencies, Dr Sellerach includes lots of information on how to eat healthily. It's a brilliant book, a real eye-opener, and I would highly recommend it. If you want something that is more solely based on nutrition, then I would recommend *The First Forty Days* by Heng Ou.

## AESTHETICS

While I really don't want aesthetics (what you look like) to be the focus of this book, how you look *can* really affect how you feel and it would be disingenuous of me to ignore this issue. As I have said before, I literally did not recognise myself in the mirror after the birth of my first child. I'm not sure how long it took me to feel like I wasn't looking at a stranger, but I do know that my relationship with my appearance has fluctuated throughout the years postpartum. I mean, I know this happens generally throughout life, but my feelings have coincided neatly with the immediate postpartum, immediately after loss and how I feel now, a few years in. Suffice to say that getting more sleep and having a modicum more time for 'self-care' or, indeed, pruning and preening, has a significant impact on how I feel about my appearance.

We know so much can change, from your hair and teeth to your tummy, posture and feet… so how do you learn to embrace your new self and feel as good as you can? Acceptance can be hard to come by if some of the changes are dramatic (as outlined by the awe-inspiring Claire Black in Chapter 8) but it is worth trying to put some time in to this. There is a quote I love from Roald Dahl, which reads *'A person who has good thoughts cannot ever be ugly. You can have a wonky nose and a crooked mouth and a double chin and stick-out teeth, but if you have good thoughts it will shine out of your face like sunbeams and you will always look lovely.'* I know that those who seem at peace, confident and accepting of themselves exude a certain *je ne sais quoi* which separates them from those of us who brood about our looks. People who feel positive about their looks have an aura that makes them more attractive, more magnetic. Look at people in your life who just have 'it' and you'll know what I mean. If your recalcitrant brain just won't let the love in, there are a couple of (non-Jedi) mind tricks that you can play on your brain to help you. Mantras and positive affirmations are proven to 'trick your brain' to boost self-esteem (there are actual studies on this – it's neuroscience, don't you know?) and smiling (no matter how fake) also tricks your brain into believing that you are genuinely feeling happy. Nothing is more attractive than a warm smile. If you've just had a night like the one I've just had (pacing the floor singing *Twinkle Twinkle Little Bloody Star* for hours), you can be forgiven for giving this a miss today.

Try to find a balance if you can. The first year with a baby is tough. Mothers often don't have the time they need to optimise their recovery and this can lead us to feeling rubbish about our bodies *and* unable to do anything about it. My advice is simply to notice what your body is doing, and whether you feel strong or weak. Your tummy and pelvic area can provoke particularly strong feelings for you and these feelings can be conflicting. You can experience gratitude, joy, pride, dislike, guilt and shame all at the same time. This area is both powerful and vulnerable and I think it is okay to treat it is such. Recognise if it makes you feel vulnerable, but perhaps also acknowledge that it was powerful enough to bring life into the world and it can become strong and powerful again to help you clear the hurdles that motherhood and ageing can present. To help you get a more realistic perspective on postpartum bodies, just take a look at the fab Fourth Trimester Bodies Project at www.4thtrimesterbodiesproject.com.

Aside from working on acceptance of your body, are there any hacks that will make small improvements aesthetically? I wouldn't personally recommend the restrictive support pants and leggings that you can get to suck your stomach in. I find them deeply uncomfortable and I think they make me look like a sausage. But lots of women do like a bit of spandex! Corsets are also making a comeback. These days they are marketed to women as 'waist trainers' (did someone press rewind to the Victorian era at some point?) but pelvic health professionals *do not* recommend them. That does not stop them being incredibly popular, with a TikTok corset challenge going viral and eliciting millions of views. I used to love a good corset, back in my board-treading days, but I can see how they could be *problematic*. If you are exerting that much pressure on your middle it's going to go up (which can restrict breathing) and down. Downward pressure on your pelvic floor is a sure-fire way to exacerbate prolapse. However, sometimes postpartum women, such as post-c-section mothers or those with significant diastasis recti, will be encouraged to use a waist support or waist trainer of some sort by a physiotherapist. Dr Sapienka, founder of FemFirst Health, says in an article for *The Independent*, 'I would not recommend anyone wearing one for weight loss or to change their body shape. For someone who has a significant diastasis recti and has been evaluated by a physical therapist who says they should wear one, then I would recommend it. For everyone else, it's a no.'

You could go for a proper bra-fitting appointment and buy some lovely new underwear that is comfortable, supportive and makes you feel like you again. You could do a wardrobe overhaul and donate the items that no longer make you feel good about yourself to charity. Create a morning routine which enables you to leave the house looking the way you want to. For me, a dedicated face-painter pre-children, this has meant radically paring down my routine so that I can leave the house on time. A very sophisticated woman I follow online states that women will always look 'done' if their eyebrows and nails are in shape. I'm inclined to agree, but I'd have to fork out monthly for beauty salon appointments to get the desired results, and my budget doesn't stretch to that at the moment. My absolute go-to for any postpartum or sleep-deprived mother is blusher. Blusher, blusher, blusher. Not so you look like Aunt Sally, or like a clown – just so you don't look like you've just been dug up. I jest. But so many people will tell you that you look radiant if you've got a bit of blusher on, and that in itself can be a real pick-me-up.

## HAIR

In Chapter 3 I explained how hair that is full and lustrous during pregnancy can be – well, the opposite – postpartum. Regrowth can also be wild. I don't remember being annoyed with my regrowth the first time around, but the second time it was coarse, grey and unruly – so, that was fun! My reaction? I dyed my hair pink to 'distract' from it. However, there are less drastic things you can do, such as continuing with the kind of high-quality supplements you probably took during pregnancy and massaging products into your scalp which will stimulate hair growth – such as nettle and rosemary oils (note, this is anecdotal, not evidence-based). Castor oil has been said to be particularly good for Afro hair and if you use weaves, braids or dreadlocks in your hairstyle, now might be a time to ask for a 'looser' style, as more pressure on the hair follicles may add to additional shedding. There are tricks you can use as your hair grows back, such as using a headband to cover the thinner areas, combing a different parting or having a deep fringe cut in. I also love a 'hack' I saw a GP mum, Dr Stephanie Jen Chyi Ooi, use on Instagram: she combed her short fly-aways down with a toothbrush covered in hairspray!

When I spoke with trichologist Sally Ann Tarver, she was sceptical about many 'hair regrowth' products and supplements. She told me that women often come to her clinic gripping a biotin supplement, but that biotin deficiency is actually said to be the rarest deficiency in the Western world. You can give yourself a head start (don't excuse the pun, it is definitely intended) by eating enough protein (hair is made of protein) and making sure your diet is nutrient-rich. You should take particular notice of your iron and vitamin B12 and vitamin D intake, and maybe consider a gentle supplement. Be aware that iron supplements can cause gastro-intestinal issues, so speak to your GP or a pharmacist first. Sally Ann advises that our hair may change a lot in the first year and regrowth can look odd, with thinning around the temples and uneven areas. Be as accepting as you can be, as this too shall pass. But, if it's getting you down, or if the hair loss is extreme or goes on for longer than 6–12 months, then it may be a good idea to see a trichologist and/or request blood tests from your GP to check for anaemia, pernicious anaemia and thyroid issues or any other deficiency. Your GP may be able to prescribe you a regrowth medication, but minoxidil (which seems to be the one that produces results) is also available over the counter. Always read the label, folks!

Sally Ann had issues with hair regrowth herself after pregnancy. She found that laser therapy worked for her, and her clients, as it stimulates regrowth. It is something that you need to do regularly for a year or so and then periodically. I had heard of laser hair removal, but was unaware that laser can also be used to encourage hair growth. It does this by stimulating blood flow to the area and therefore stimulating the follicles for hair growth. Research on the topic is mixed, and sometimes clouded by being too closely associated with the manufacturers, but the overall picture is largely positive. Sally Ann has found that it has restored her hair to its pre-pregnancy state. However, it is not suitable for pregnant women, breastfeeding women or those taking photo-sensitive drugs. Efficacy aside, laser therapy is likely out of reach for many of us, or an avenue we are not keen to pursue – so what else can we do? Remember that in general relatively small amounts of hair are lost and in most cases your hair will be back to normal within a few months or a year without you having to make any effort at all.

Sally Ann does not rate caffeine shampoos particularly highly, but she does have some other tips which could help. If you have dark hair, then Nanogen hair fibres shaken into the hair will visually bolster thinning hair. Also, having your hair coloured makes it swell, which can give the impression of increased volume. Dry shampoo can also add volume to flat or fine hair. There are many other ideas out there, from micro-needling to platelet-rich plasma treatment, but proceed with caution and patience, as in the vast majority of cases hair worries are a short-term bugbear.

## SKIN

When my skin went dry and bumpy, about five months postpartum, I went back to two things I was doing in the immediate postnatal period, when my skin was clear and glowy. One was drinking *loads* of water, and the second was taking probiotics. I am not the only one who swears by these for better skin. British actress and new mum Jodie Turner-Smith also recently credited probiotics for helping postpartum acne. A third thing I did was to start using a (breastfeeding friendly!) acid on my face. The idea of using anything with the word acid in it used to make me recoil, but a little bit of low grade BHA was all I needed. I actually think the water and the probiotics would have worked without the acid, but I am now in my 40s and have started spending the equivalent of mortgage payments every month on skincare in a bid to regain a little of the flush of youth I had before I had kids! It pays to do your research on skincare products, as many will promise you the earth. Trusted sources, such as Caroline Hirons and Skin Nerds (who do online consultations), are worth looking at.

*Loose skin.* This might be something you need to try to learn to love. Surgery can be indicated in extreme cases, but it really is a last resort. Micro-needling has been mooted as a potential aid in increasing collagen production and the appearance of the skin, but there are no studies to support this. I haven't tried it myself so I am not endorsing it! As with most things that people want to sell us: if it's a problem for you then absolutely seek out a solution – but if it isn't, don't let our modern consumerist/perfectionist society tell you there's something wrong when there isn't. The real keys for optimum skin health are hydration and nutrition. You may not be able to get rid of all the baggy skin, but you can improve its appearance by building lean muscle underneath to increase the appearance of tautness – as well as keeping skin looking healthy through being hydrated and getting enough protein and vitamins such as vitamin E and vitamin C.

*Dry skin.* A few things that can help are: using non-perfumed, alcohol-free, hypo-allergenic products; making sure your shower or bath is not too hot and you don't stay in too long (chance would be a fine thing); applying a body oil in the shower while your body is wet to lock in the moisture; and ensuring you are getting enough healthy fats (nuts, seeds, avocados, olive oil) in your diet. Even now, when I can, I apply a body oil all over before I get into the bath or shower. The water will not take all the oil off, so this allows me to get some much-needed moisture on to my skin. Once you're out of the bath or shower, you can often feel back 'on duty' again, and you run out of time for moisturising.

**Spots.** Double cleansing (cleansing twice, first with a rich cream and then something lighter, like a milk – but never anything foaming) appears to be the way forward. Some acids can help bumpy skin, but choose your products carefully. Also, with absolutely nothing to back this up, apart from my own experience, I will suggest applying some breastmilk to any inflamed or spotty skin. It is both soothing and antibacterial so worth a shot! For actual expert skin tips, I highly recommend following the aforementioned Caroline Hirons on social media or buying her (pretty comprehensive) book *Skin Care*. If your skin does not clear up, your GP can refer you to a dermatologist.

**Melasma.** Use your SPF, protect your skin from the sun – and it should settle down.

Jennifer Rock, founder of Skin Nerds, has this to say – which I fully agree with (your skin being your biggest organ, and all that): 'We can often feel guilty – especially those with small children – about investing in our skin. I really don't believe having a cleanser, a serum and an SPF is about anything more than minding an organ – having the core parts of skincare right is something we all deserve.'

## LOOK AFTER YOUR FEET

Your poor tootsies. They put up with a lot from us, and they often get very little TLC in return. After the weight gain and hormonal shifts of pregnancy, it is important to take some time to look after your feet. First, give them a break. Walk around barefoot when you can and, when wearing shoes, try not to squeeze them Ugly-Sister-like into shoes which are now too small. If you have fallen arches that are bothersome, it might be worth getting an arch support to make walking more comfortable. Also, giving yourself a foot massage and stretch will really help you to rebalance. You can lace your fingers between your toes and make sure your toes are really spread out and give them a vigorous rub and kneading motion. Likewise, rolling a ball (a children's bouncy ball is perfect) under your foot can feel heavenly (in an 'ooof' kind of way) as you release all of that pent-up stress on your foot. The one-legged balance suggested in the previous chapter can also really help with strengthening the whole area of the foot, ankle and calf, to give you more support. This is because it helps engage a set of muscles that run along the shins and calves and to the inside of the foot. Do not worry if you wobble: the wobbling encourages these muscles to activate. If you're a yoga fan, then the Tree Pose will also do this.

## MAKE FRIENDS WITH YOUR BATHROOM

If you have a male partner, you may find (incoming: huge generalisation but based on *a lot* of real-time data/gossip) that the bathroom can be occupied for long stretches of time. It's time to take a leaf out of the Dad Handbook here. Your bathroom may be the only place where you can lock the door and concentrate on yourself – for months (or years!). I chortled in recognition when I listened to Victoria Maw on the Postnatal FAQ podcast recount how she often unrolls her yoga mat and engages in some light stretching during her 'toilet trips'. I have been known to do a whole body workout, while covered in body oil, hair mask and face mask, before a shower. Then I do my pelvic floor exercises in the shower and top it all off with a full on showtunes singing session to release tension and get my diaphragm moving (flexibility in the diaphragm is important for core and pelvic health/ strength). Last but not least, I indulge in a spot of Wim-Hof*-lite cold water therapy, which is said to boost immunity and mood, among other things. All of this takes about 20 minutes. Reclaim some time. Get thee to the bathroom.

---

* Wim Hof is a Dutch motivational speaker and 'extreme' athlete who promotes the health benefits of cold water showers and swimming.

# CHAPTER 7

# BUMPS IN THE ROAD

I hope you sail through pregnancy, birth and postpartum. I hope you only experience a fraction of the symptoms and conditions mentioned in previous chapters. I hope you and your babies are supported to thrive.

I know, however, that life can throw curveballs. And, just as it's wholly unrealistic when fairy tales end with that 'and they lived happily ever after' shtick, you generally don't go riding off into the sunset on a unicorn once your baby arrives. You're kind of in it for the long haul. And that can mean all sorts of different things, for all sorts of different people. In this chapter we will cover what postpartum (both immediate and longer term) can look like for those with physical complications, disabilities, chronic conditions, those from minority or marginalised backgrounds and those who have experienced loss or had a baby in NICU (neonatal intensive care unit), as well as common postnatal health issues that can become serious. While I was keen to cover as many different facets of postpartum as possible, this is not in any way exhaustive. All of the added layers of complexity that I write about briefly here deserve much more time and detail, so please do refer to the resources at the end of the book for more thorough information.

## WHEN THINGS DON'T GO TO PLAN

I had my entire postnatal period planned. Reader, I *did* my postnatal plan. I had a local friend, who is a reiki healer, lined up to assist me in a doula-type role. I had formed a WhatsApp group of close local friends to help me with things like the school run for my eldest. I had batch cooked. I was ready to call on people for help. But, then, BAM! Two weeks after baby no.2 arrived, the UK went into lockdown – meaning my eldest was sent home from school (indefinitely), nobody was allowed to visit, and shops began to run low on supplies like toilet roll, bread, and nappies. Both my husband and my eldest son contracted Covid-19 – which turned into long Covid (similar to the condition ME) for my husband. To say this was a testing time is an understatement. My 'discharge' visit from my midwife had her standing outside our porch (masked up) as my husband and I weighed our new baby in the hallway. My son had tongue-tie and cow's milk protein allergy. I was recovering from a c-section. All my carefully laid plans went up in a puff of smoke. As they did for most people at this time. I felt so keenly for first-time mothers. I remembered how hard it was. But this was not my first rodeo. And it is amazing how we adapt. It was not the postpartum period I hoped for. It was not conducive to rest and recuperation. But we survived. Without everything that I am advocating for in this book – rest, nurturing, good follow-up care, the chance for respite – we still managed. I even – among the rubble – have some lovely memories of this time.

Life will throw hard stuff at us. Hopefully for you this will not be a full-blown pandemic, but if other life-altering challenges come at you postpartum – know that you can overcome them. We women, birthing people, humans, are resilient. If you can't do some of – or anything – this book recommends you will still be okay. Life isn't perfect and things do not always go to plan. If life becomes difficult for other reasons after your birth, it is even more important to reach out. There will always be people who are going through, or have been through, similar. There are always stories of triumph over adversity and there is no reason why yours can't be one of them.

## PELVIC ISSUES

While most pelvic issues will resolve with time and care, sometimes they can persist and this can be incredibly emotionally draining. If you suffered a third- or fourth-degree tear, or a significant levator ani injury, you may have a steeper mountain to climb to fully heal. If you have tried a women's health physio, and retraining your pelvic floor, and you are still experiencing pain, discomfort, prolapse or continence issues, it may be that you will need to have a conversation about other treatment options, including surgery.

There are many different types of surgery for prolapse. 'Mesh' was widely utilised until very recently, when women who had been severely injured or disabled as a result of using it campaigned for a ban or tighter legislation. Now 'native tissue' (using your own tissue) is more prevalent. Ongoing scrutiny of mesh implants continues, as a recent paper states: 'Meshes have been used very effectively in vaginal surgery. As prolapse is a very common problem, we need effective and resilient surgical techniques with a low risk profile'.[51] What they are saying is that while many women benefitted from mesh, there need to be more robust safety measures, as we cannot risk some women being worse off after their surgery than they were before they had it.

Surgery is sometimes considered for continence issues, but for urinary incontinence (UI) it is advisable to work with a good physio, or team of physios, first as advances are constantly being made in how to improve UI. Physio may also help with faecal incontinence, but from what I've read, this is sometimes a tall order. With that in mind, the NHS suggests four other potential options: a sphincteroplasty operation (to repair anal sphincter muscle); injections with a bulking agent such as silicone to make the muscle stronger; sacral nerve stimulation (where a small electronic device is placed under your skin to help your muscles and nerves work better); or (last resort) a colostomy bag (this is where your bowel is diverted through a hole made in your abdomen so that faeces can be collected in a bag). If the last option seems scary to you, and it's something you feel might be in your future, do take a look at 'colostomummy' online for support. Sacral nerve stimulation is also sometimes used for urinary issues such as an 'overactive bladder'.

One further option for continence issues is percutaneous tibial nerve stimulation (PTNS), which is a newer therapy and can be used for both bladder and bowel issues. PTNS is minimally invasive, and also stimulates the sacral nerve, which regulates bowel function. It is an outpatient procedure, rather than an operation, but it may take three months to complete a course of treatment. Research is patchier on the efficacy of this versus sacral nerve stimulation (which is an operation requiring recovery time).

Most health practitioners I have spoken to have said that surgery is never a first line response. There are always other, less invasive treatments you can try first and, as more is understood about women's health and healing after birth, and more advances are made, surgery can often wait, if it is needed at all.

This is an emotive issue, so try to ensure you have decent support (if talking with family members or friends is too difficult, do engage with the Birth Trauma Association or MASIC Foundation). Always discuss all of your options fully, and get a second opinion if you can. You will see from the next chapter that surgery, if needed, needn't be too alarming and can help you regain confidence and a sense of getting your life back.

## POSTPARTUM THYROIDITIS

Postpartum thyroiditis is a condition that affects roughly 5–10% of women after pregnancy, and usually occurs within a year after birth. The thyroid is a small, butterfly-shaped gland at the base of the neck and secretes thyroid hormones which regulate heart, muscle and digestive function, brain development and bone maintenance. Symptoms of hyperthyroidism (too much thyroid hormone in the bloodstream) and hypothyroidism (too little thyroid in the bloodstream) can mimic common postnatal symptoms, so you need a blood test to determine if a malfunctioning thyroid is the cause. Symptoms of a thyroid issue can include: fatigue, fast or irregular heartbeat, sweating, either losing or gaining weight with no real reason, anxiety, hair loss, sensitivity to temperature fluctuations, sluggish bowels, and dry/brittle nails. Jenny Allen, who campaigns for greater awareness of this condition, explained how, for her, it was like a 'rollercoaster', with going from feeling irritable with racing thoughts, to feeling extreme fatigue and depression. If you are struggling with all of this and you go for a thyroid test and it comes back 'normal' it may be worth following up privately, if you can afford it, as NHS tests can be limited. As nutritionist Jo Sharp says, in the NHS you are either 'sick' or 'well' and it doesn't account for those that fall between these spheres. There are more conclusive thyroid tests available, and it is worth exploring.

## PUDENDAL NEURALGIA

This painful condition can sometimes be caused by childbirth.

Pudendal neuralgia causes pain or numbness in the pelvic area and symptoms can include painful sex, a prickling or burning sensation around any part of your undercarriage and a feeling of swelling on the perineum, increased urination and a deep pelvic pain – among others. Treatment may include specialist painkillers for nerve pain, physiotherapy, nerve stimulation and injectable steroids. Sometimes surgery to remove tissue might be performed. My research shows me that some sufferers use other 'complementary' therapies such as acupuncture and osteopathy to help with the pain.

## VULVODYNIA

Vulvodynia is persistent, 'unexplained' pain (including a burning or stinging sensation) and/or discomfort in the vulva. It is thought to be caused by a potential 'excess' of nerve endings in the vulval area which have been damaged. Although it can last a long time, it can also go away 'on its own'. All of the 'normal' after-effects of childbirth can further irritate those who suffer with vulvodynia and, sometimes, it only starts after childbirth. Your vulva will not look any different. Treatments vary and can include advice on gentle hygiene practices (no harsh chemicals or douches), using correct lubrication, using lidocaine numbing cream if you wish to resume sex, physiotherapy, the use of vaginal dilators, Botox to block the release of pain signals and psychosexual counselling (although this last one may pertain more to those who suffer with vaginismus – an involuntary muscle spasm which makes sexual touch and intercourse painful or impossible – as it is most often coupled with anxiety around sex).

## ENDOMETRIOSIS IN CAESAREAN SCARS

Endometriosis is a condition where tissue similar to the lining of the womb starts to grow in other places, such as the ovaries and fallopian tubes. It is fairly common (affecting 10% of women worldwide) and can be very painful and distressing. It is a widespread and complex condition. There is evidence that pregnancy itself can help ease the symptoms of endometriosis but there have not been any studies on how endometriosis 'behaves' after pregnancy. However, a study in Sweden in 2013 found that giving birth via caesarean section slightly increased the risk of developing endometriosis. Researchers noted that 'In addition to the recognised risk of scar endometrioma, we found an association between caesarean section and general pelvic endometriosis.'[52] Sometimes your period will affect how the scar feels: 'Scar endometriosis has also been described as a painful swelling of the scar that is worse during menses (menstruation)'.[53] If it is particularly bad, you may be a candidate for surgery to get rid of the excess endometrial-like tissue.

## DIABETES (FOLLOWING GESTATIONAL DIABETES)

Gestational diabetes is a common (16%[54] of pregnant women develop GD) temporary condition which raises your blood sugar levels during pregnancy. A hormone made by the placenta prevents your body from using insulin effectively. It is not clear why some women develop gestational diabetes and others don't, but risk factors include being overweight and having diabetes in the family. It can be miserable getting through pregnancy with diabetes, with all of the extra monitoring, the strict diet and the drugs, let alone feeling poorly on top of it. It is so great to have that light at the end of the tunnel that when baby comes earthside, quickly followed by that naughty placenta, you will (most likely) be free of the condition. I, for one (and I am *not* condoning this at all) had a ginormous Toblerone packed in my hospital bag and dispatched it *tout de suite* once I'd given birth. Unfortunately (and I am so sorry to be the Haribo-hiding harbinger of doom), you are at a significantly increased risk of developing Type 2 diabetes if you have experienced gestational diabetes. It sucks. And not in a rhubarb and custard boiled sweet way. More in a sucking on a wasp kinda way.

It is thought that roughly over half of women who present with gestational diabetes will go on to develop Type 2 diabetes. Although gestational diabetes normally disappears as soon as the baby is born, you should be invited to the GP surgery for a blood test at between six weeks and 13 weeks, and then every year thereafter to check your blood sugar levels. It can be worrying to hear these statistics and have these tests. I know as I had gestational diabetes with both of my full-term pregnancies. Your risk of developing Type 2 diabetes is compounded by age (being over 40), race/ethnicity (being from Black African, African Caribbean and South Asian backgrounds), having a family member with Type 2 diabetes, having polycystic ovarian syndrome, smoking and being overweight. Having had gestational diabetes in pregnancy also increases your risk of cardiovascular disorders, renal disorders, nerve, and eye issues.[55] Having gestational diabetes once also increases your risk of developing it in subsequent pregnancies. Medical professionals will encourage you to follow a balanced diet, try and keep within a healthy weight for your frame, quit smoking and undertake adequate exercise.

## HYPERTENSION (FOLLOWING PRE-ECLAMPSIA)

High blood pressure, also known as 'hypertension,' means that the blood pressure in the arteries is persistently elevated. It is common in pregnancy – affecting 3–7%[56] of pregnant women – and can be related to a pre-existing condition or the condition pre-eclampsia.

If you had high blood pressure before you became pregnant, or had blood pressure problems in your last pregnancy, you are at an increased risk of similar complications in future pregnancies. The risk of complications in any future pregnancies depends on how severe your problem was and how many weeks pregnant you were when the high blood pressure started. The effect tends to occur later in the next pregnancy, but it can still be severe.

This next bit is a bit shocking, so brace yourself: a recent study found that the risk of developing a serious heart and circulatory condition increased by 45% if a woman had high blood pressure during pregnancy, and by nearly 70% if you had pre-eclampsia, compared to those who had normal blood pressure during pregnancy.[57] While these statistics are alarming, there are measures you can take, so bear with. Firstly, do not berate yourself: you cannot go back in time and change anything. Start where you are and work from there. Even if you could have changed anything, there are a variety of reasons high blood pressure occurs, including: genetics, hormones, age, diabetes, and sleep issues. Black ethnicity is also a risk factor, as is being pregnant with multiples. You have the facts and stats, so what now? Be proactive in managing your health, which means keeping an eye on your blood pressure from now on and seeking means to manage it for the long term – which could include: ensuring you visit your GP annually for a blood pressure check, even if it has returned to normal after pregnancy; maintaining a healthy weight and looking to reduce salt and 'bad' fats (we need some fat in our diet, but go sparingly with things like pies, sausages, cream and butter); quitting smoking (smoking narrows blood vessels, making it easier for fat to clog arteries); limiting alcohol and caffeine; and staying as active as you can.

## CHRONIC CONDITIONS AND DISABILITIES

If I were to try to chronicle every health condition we could suffer with, and how to manage it in the postnatal period, I would probably be writing forever – this book would never be published, and you'd never read it. Therefore, my plea to you is: if you are living with a long-term health condition, please be aware that pregnancy can exacerbate symptoms and it is *perfectly* okay to seek as much help and support as possible. As well as speaking to your healthcare providers, the internet is often a wonderful resource when it comes to finding communities supporting one another with health conditions and worries.

One area where women are over-represented in health conditions is autoimmune disorders. Autoimmune diseases affect around 8% of our population, and a whopping 78%[58] of these are women. This can be anything from something as rare as Bechet's disease (a multi-system inflammatory disorder) to more commonly recognised diseases such as rheumatoid arthritis. I spoke to rheumatologist Dr Iona Thorne, who has a specialist interest in obstetrics. She told me that while autoimmune conditions can improve – or be almost sent into remission during pregnancy, as the immune system is suppressed – there can be a 'rebound' postnatally. This normally happens between 8–16 weeks postnatally as hormones rebalance and the immune system returns to normal. This is backed up by the experience of my friend Rachael, a nurse and mum of two in Wales, who suffers with Bechet's. 'I blossomed, bloomed and bounced through my pregnancy. My disease went into remission and even resolved an ongoing symptom completely. Hurrah for pregnancy hormones! My rheumatologist said she wished she could bottle the hormones for me. There was even hope that I would remain in remission for up to a year after giving birth – it has been known to happen in other autoimmune diseases'. Unfortunately for Rachael this wasn't the case, and her disease began to flare again at the end of her pregnancy. Rachael found the postpartum period extremely difficult as her disease flared aggressively as she battled sleep deprivation and trying to learn to breastfeed. Rachael was desperate to breastfeed, but Bechet's made this particularly difficult as her body was already trying to heal from the exertion of labour and the resurfacing of inflammation: 'My consultant was not surprised to hear my nipples were in shreds and that my milk supply was insufficient. Having a chronic disease puts a real strain on your body. The effort of producing milk was not a priority for a body raging with inflammation. I had to stop breastfeeding/expressing to go back on infliximab (a 'biological' therapy used for autoimmune conditions) and needed to be fully healed. It's never easy making decisions that are due to a disease; it doesn't feel like a choice, and you feel so let down by a body that's meant to protect you, not attack you.' Rachael also struggled with recurrent mastitis, which was a big problem as the immune-suppressing drugs she needed to take would make her more susceptible to sepsis.

Reading Rachael's heart-breaking account of not just her first pregnancy, but her second (which was much more difficult), brought home to me how very, very difficult coping with the postpartum period is when you are also living with a chronic disease or condition. It also became clear how essential it is to have a support system in place in advance – from your consultant, your midwife/obstetrician and GP through to family, friends, and your community. Iona stressed to me that her most pertinent advice would be to have pre-planned reviews and assessments with your healthcare advisors, as the system is not yet joined up or progressive enough to give women with these types of complications the timely care they need. Iona impressed on me that women must advocate for themselves and flag any issues throughout pregnancy, as well as setting up appointments in advance. As a mother of young children herself, she knows that in the postpartum period a new mother will be too tired and distracted to begin thinking about making more health appointments. She is also adamant that mothers should discuss contraception at the earliest opportunity, as someone with an autoimmune condition must try to have enough of a gap between pregnancies to allow their body to recover and gain strength.

With regards to a support network, Rachael explains that she has learnt that this is key to getting through not just the hard times, but also everyday life with a rare disease: 'I'm not great at asking for help but I'm getting better. I no longer refuse friends' offers of a cooked meal to put in the freezer or a catch up – that usually means I'm in tears. I'm slowly learning that I have a village of people around me, and that motherhood with a disease to fight as well is bloody hard, but it needn't be a fight you face alone.'

Iona also pointed out that the postpartum period is not just a time when autoimmune conditions flare, but also when they surface for the first time. Several studies have shown that women are at increased risk of developing autoimmune conditions in pregnancy or postnatally, including a 1999 study[59] which states, 'We found that postpartum onset of rheumatoid arthritis was found in 0.08% of women in the general population and could be partially predicted by measuring rheumatoid factors in early pregnancy. There are several case reports of other autoimmune diseases that develop after delivery: postpartum renal failure or postdelivery haemolytic-uremic syndrome, postpartum idiopathic polymyositis, postpartum syndrome with antiphospholipid antibodies, postpartum autoimmune myocarditis. Many other possible postpartum autoimmune diseases are still unexplored.' One woman who experienced postpartum onset of an autoimmune condition is writer and wedding celebrant Keli Tomlin, who lives in Glossop with her seven-year-old son. After a long, arduous birth, which Keli found traumatic, she began to feel extreme fatigue and a low mood. She put this down to the usual strains of new motherhood initially, but her health declined gradually over two years, to a point where she could not climb the stairs in her own home as her muscles had weakened so much and she was so tired. Up until this point, doctors had dismissed her health concerns as being tied up with her 'extended breastfeeding'. However, it was a different hormonal imbalance (not oestrogen) that was the source of her feeling 'like I was fading.' Eventually, it was a summer tan that didn't fade in the winter that alerted a GP to refer Keli to an endocrinologist who tested her for Addison's disease (a rare disorder of the adrenal glands). Getting the diagnosis, and subsequent medication, two years after first presenting with symptoms, was a huge relief for Keli. She says 'Within two weeks,

I was like a different person. It was like coming back from the dead.' She tells me that, although it is a balance to get her medication levels correct, she feels 'well' and can do everything in her life that she would like to. She does feel she missed out on the first two years of her son's life though, as she did not have the energy levels to properly adapt and enjoy new motherhood. She had felt like she 'just wasn't cut out to be a mum'. Keli is certain that the stress of her labour was what triggered the issues with her adrenal glands, although there is currently no research that could back this up. She implores other mothers not to feel ashamed if they are not coping, and to reach out for help. One positive that came out of all of this for Keli is that she now recognises more about what she needs to thrive, and 'gives this to herself'.

Dr Iona Thorne told me that if you 'do not feel right,' then not to just dismiss it, go and see a health professional. You know your body better than anyone. It is certainly hard in the initial postpartum period to work out what is normal and what isn't, but if you are worried – there is no harm in chatting through any worries with your GP.

Another mother who struggled with chronic health issues after childbirth is Sharmika Dockery. Sharmika has shared her full story via the campaigning platform 'Five x More',[60] which highlights the disparities between maternal outcomes for black and white women in the UK, and campaigns for change. We spoke about Sharmika's postpartum journey and how difficult she has found it over the last seven years to get a proper diagnosis and deal with pain relief. Sharmika lives with constant pain and mobility issues, believed to have been caused by a missed retained placenta, and subsequent surgeries, after the birth of her son Riley when she was just 17. The main barrier to healing that Sharmika has found is being listened to and believed. In fact, in early appointments, she found that her own GP had suggested midwives keep an eye on her parenting and she found that this became the focus, and not the pain and excessive sweating that turned out to be due to the retained placenta tissue. Sharmika has had a number of operations and procedures to try and get to the root of her ongoing pain and mobility issues but feels that a full explanation is yet to be discovered. We spoke about what has made her journey easier and she told me that she is a huge fan of meditation and credits this with helping her remain calm during days with 'flare-ups.' She also speaks passionately about how reaching out to others going through the same, or similar, experiences has helped her feel less isolated. Under the moniker @spooniemama_x, Sharmika connects with other parents, and individuals, who class themselves as 'spoonies'. Spoonie is a term coined by a chronic illness blogger, Christine Miserandino, who used spoons to demonstrate how much energy a person with a chronic illness has each day, and how much is used up doing simple tasks like washing or getting dressed. Sharmika has gone further than documenting her own struggles to create a wider network; she has set up an online community called Beyond Strength, which has allowed parents with disabilities and long-term health conditions to connect and support each other. Sharmika is keen that this be replicated 'IRL' (in real life) and so is building an app that will reproduce this community and help create local 'village-like' support networks. In addition to this, Sharmika's journey took a real turn when she moved hospitals and involved a patient advocate organisation called Voice Ability. Voice Ability provided an advocate to attend Sharmika's appointments with her and ensure she was being listened to and taken seriously. They actually involved someone from the board of the hospital trust, at which point progress with referrals and diagnosis was speeded up.

It shouldn't have to be this way. Sharmika's voice should have been respected and listened to years before, but it is helpful to know there are organisations like this out there to help if you are feeling dismissed and struggling to get the treatment you need. There is still a long way to go, not just for Sharmika, but for postpartum women in general, to truly be heard and cared for as they need to be, but organisations like this – and communities like Sharmika's – are beginning to make a difference.

Dr Sally Pezaro, a midwife and academic, has been doing fascinating work in the area of Ehlers-Danlos syndrome (EDS) and hypermobility, and the effects of these conditions on pregnancy, birth and postpartum. It is estimated that 1 in 20 pregnant women have EDS,[61] although it is currently underdiagnosed. As well as joint hypermobility, the condition can cause all manner of other symptoms such as migraine, gastro-intestinal issues, or cardiovascular problems.

Although EDS can potentially cause some issues in pregnancy, it is believed that pregnancy is generally 'well tolerated' in people with hypermobile EDS(hEDS) or hypermobility spectrum disorder (HSD). However, it is absolutely worth talking with your care team about the condition and how to manage labour and birth, as some considerations need to be addressed (such as anaesthesia and pain relief, for example). Postpartum, hypermobility or EDS is known to be the root of some issues, and to increase the likelihood of some adverse outcomes, which is why Dr Pezaro is raising awareness of the condition, its prevalence, and manifestations. She is particularly keen that midwives become aware of the conditions, as it can positively inform practice. Some issues that women with hEDS/HSD (whether diagnosed or not) may be more susceptible to are wound dehiscence (breakdown of the wound), prolapse, persistent pelvic girdle pain, coccyx dislocation and haemorrhage – among others. Consideration of potential increased joint laxity (whereby the pregnancy hormones exacerbate a pre-existing condition like hypermobility) could help you plan around carrying 'your new load' as it grows, ensuring you are taking extra precautions not to dislocate or put more stress on unstable joints. Or you might consider a support belt to help keep your pelvis more stable in the weeks following the birth. Pelvic floor expert Marianne Ryan enthuses about these in her book *Baby Bod*. One American study showed that women with a diagnosis of EDS generally needed a longer stay in hospital post-birth (although the study was limited by the fact that they didn't differentiate between the 14+ different sub-types of the syndrome), so it might be worth noting this so that your hospital bag is adequate, and you can mentally prepare yourself.

## DISABILITY

In 2018 Birthrights, a charity that promotes human rights in childbirth, commissioned a survey into the experiences of women and birthing people with disabilities. As well as finding that individualised care and support were thin on the ground throughout pregnancy, the personal accounts from these women showed a lack of understanding of how disability can affect the postpartum period. Postnatal wards, in particular, were flagged as being inaccessible and postnatal care in general was where rates of satisfaction were lowest. I spoke with the incredibly sunny (don't worry, I'm not going to call you an inspiration, Kara!) @happy_para_mum to get a little more insight into the additional issues that disability can throw at women postpartum. Kara Scott hails from Yorkshire and is on a mission to show what is possible as a disabled mother of two. She runs an Instagram account whereby she chronicles her day-to-day life (including going on a TV gameshow) with her family. Kara discovered she was pregnant with her second child shortly after finding out that her condition, transverse myelitis, had caused paralysis from T5 (just below the ribs) downwards. Kara spoke with me about how she found pregnancy hard and was unable to feel her baby move, and so she worried about the bond. Once Winnie arrived, however, she was completely besotted and set about adapting to her new life. The initial postpartum period did throw up some issues, as, although she could not feel pain from her c-section due to the paralysis, she found the postnatal ward a challenge. 'They were very nice, and so busy, but there was no awareness of how to deal with someone in a wheelchair, or how someone with a spinal cord injury needs assistance with going to the toilet.' Kara ended up with a compacted bowel and just wanted to go home so that she and her husband could manage her bowel care properly themselves. Kara has adapted impressively to the new challenges, both physical and mental, that motherhood and disability have brought. She shares how she deals with everyday issues and the more difficult times, such as illness and operations, on a very upbeat and aesthetically beautiful Instagram feed. I do suggest you follow her, whether you have a disability or not, as you can't help but fall in love with her a bit. It clearly happened to Jimmy Carr too, as after she appeared on his game show, he invited her out to dinner. When I asked Kara for her advice for other disabled mothers, she told me this, 'Don't beat yourself up because you're not doing it like everyone else. And don't be swayed by other people telling you how to be a mum. They don't have to adapt like you do. Also, people are quite willing to help so don't berate yourself for asking for help if you need it.'

## BEING FROM A MINORITY ETHNIC GROUP

You may have noticed when reading this book that some of the more adverse outcomes can be more prevalent in black women, and women from other 'minority ethnic' groups. Pregnancy can be a nervous enough time as it is, without glaring statistics such as those from the MBRRACE[62] report* and additional worries about postpartum health playing on your mind. Along with all of the other parts of this chapter, maternal health for women from black and brown communities deserves a book (books!) all to itself. As a white woman, I have no knowledge of what it feels like to go through pregnancy, birth and postpartum as a woman of colour. What I do know, is that such are the disparities between outcomes for black and white women (and neonates) highlighted by reports from MBRRACE, that an All-Party Parliamentary Group (APPG) has recently been formed to address these issues. Alongside campaigns run by women from these communities, it seems that finally these disparities might begin to be addressed. One thing that crops up repeatedly is susceptibility to hypertension (high blood pressure) and Type 2 diabetes among people from black and South Asian backgrounds. These two conditions can be exacerbated in pregnancy and need to be monitored carefully postpartum. The reasons why these diseases are more prevalent in black and ethnic minority groups are not yet well researched, but this sentence from a Kings Fund report[63] sums up some of the interacting factors: *Unpicking the causes of ethnic inequalities in health is difficult. Available evidence suggests a complex interplay of deprivation, environmental, physiological, behavioural, and cultural factors. Ethnic minority groups are disproportionately affected by socio-economic deprivation, a key determinant of health status. This is driven by a wider social context in which structural racism can reinforce inequalities among ethnic groups, for example in housing, employment, and the criminal justice system, which in turn can have a negative impact on their health. Evidence shows that racism and discrimination can also have a negative impact on the physical and mental health of people from ethnic minority groups.*

---

* The most recent MBRRACE report shows that shows the disparity in maternal mortality rates between women from black and Asian aggregated ethnic groups and White women remains more than four times higher for black women, two times higher for mixed ethnicity women and almost twice as high for Asian women.

It is not just about genetics and social aspects though: there is a clear need for a fundamental shift within the healthcare system to ensure all women are listened to and treated equally. If you are active on social media, or an avid reader, you may have read some accounts from black women about their treatment within a maternity setting, with perhaps the most 'accessible' (due to her huge platform) being tennis champion Serena Williams, whose fears about suffering with a pulmonary embolism were originally erroneously dismissed by her nurse. Serena has stated 'I think there's a lot of pre-judging, absolutely, that definitely goes on. And it needs to be spoken about, it needs to be addressed.' In the UK, author Candice Brathwaite paints a similarly stark picture in her book *I Am Not Your Baby Mother*, stating 'I had not been cared for, let alone listened to. How there was this general expectation – even from health care providers who looked like me – for me to be strong and silent'. Suffice to say, big changes need to occur and thanks to the efforts of people like birth worker Mars Lord, and the Association of South Asian Midwives, shifts are happening. We can all start by bearing witness to what black and brown women are experiencing. If you are a woman of colour, and the findings from the MBRRACE report concern you, there are places you can reach out to – including the FivexMore organisation and The Motherhood Group. Many women, and allies, are rising up to provide better care and support to mitigate against adverse outcomes. And please don't forget, that while the statistics are alarming, the UK is still one of the safest places in the world to give birth.

When I spoke with Sabah Quereshi,* a mother of two from the South Asian community, she made it clear to me that her postpartum healing journey was hampered by feeling dismissed and disbelieved by medical professionals, which she partly puts down to her ethnic origin. Her fight to be heard started in labour and by the time she was postpartum she was finding it hard to summon the energy to make her voice heard. As she lay in the labour ward, being stitched by someone she did not have confidence in, she feels she was subjected to assertions (such as this not being her last child, as it was her second girl) that were founded on her being of South Asian origin. Now eight months postpartum, she has had numerous health appointments

---

* Not her real name

to help her heal from a misdiagnosed and poorly repaired perineal tear and has had her mental health questioned for not wanting more invasive physical examinations. Sabah believes that conscious or unconscious bias has played a part in some of her interactions with health professionals. She feels that as a woman (and particularly as a South Asian woman), you are meant be quiet and accepting both of what is 'done' to your body, and any ramifications, and when you don't subscribe to this, and fight for yourself, you are deemed a nuisance or even emotionally imbalanced. Sabah feels this extends beyond the health sector, and she knows first-hand how hard it is to suffer with a birth injury within a community where people do not talk about such things. She told me that not even her own mother knows how difficult her postpartum experience has been as 'there will be an air of superstition or karma, as if you did something to bring this on yourself.' Pooja Shah, a writer in New York, notes in an article for *Vice*[64] that this tendency to keep quiet about trauma extends to the emotional fall-out from birth and subsequent postnatal depression. Sabah says she feels 'mentally strong', but she is still on her healing journey, and although things began to improve from five months postpartum, she still deals with pain and continence issues daily. Sabah is determined to get to the root of her issues and heal to a point where she can enjoy life with her husband and daughters. She has a dogged determination, despite setbacks, and is keen that women, from all backgrounds, don't stop fighting to be heard. This can be exhausting when you are in pain, but Sabah knows that she sometimes needs to keep chasing referrals and appointments in order to get her closer to her goal of returning to a more comfortable physical state.

Sabah and I spoke about what a difference it would make if she could be more open and if she had more support and understanding, both from her community and the health service, and she is acutely aware that women from a similar background who perhaps do not have the same level of education or confidence may be really struggling mentally as well as physically. I spoke with Sundas Khalid from the South Asian Midwives Association, and she recognises the scenario faced by Sabah very well (of experiencing racism within the maternity setting and struggling with being open in her own community). Sundas is clear that there is a lot of work to be done with regards to healthcare equality and cultural change, but things *are* changing: 'Six years ago, I would never have been able to have a conversation with my family about birth, but now, because of my training, knowledge and experience, we are so much more open. Conversations are happening and women do want to know about what is happening to them in pregnancy and birth, they want that knowledge. They are not "hard to reach" as everyone says, we just need to find different ways to reach them.' Sundas was a delight to talk to, so passionate about her work and her community. She was just about to begin work on a summit to celebrate excellence for brown and black birth workers, called 'Through the Dark Lens,' which sounded all kinds of amazing. If you are reading this and feel let down by the health service, or isolated within your community, know that there are people working tirelessly for change and there are organisations you can reach out to.

## OLDER MUMS

Hello fellow geriatric mothers (waves)…sorry, I had to. That term, though! Folks, (paging – yes, this is irony – all doctors/nurses) it's *time to change* this language. As well as other redundant, old-fashioned, misogynistic, and plain old *rude* terminology,* it's time to bin this phrase. However, it turns out that being an older mum can present you with a few more bumps than the one protruding from your belly.

While researching this book, it became clear that many pregnancy and postpartum difficulties can be exacerbated by being more advanced in age. Older mothers can be at increased risk of 'adverse outcomes' such as diabetes, hypertension and pelvic floor issues. This is such a tricky area to address because the reasons women are having babies later are multiple and there is a balance to be struck when reporting on the increase in any risks. I had my first child at 34 and my second at 39 and as an 'older mum', I can say that creating a financially and emotionally secure base from which to start a family was crucial for me (okay, okay as well as something of a Peter Pan

---

* See the Peanut app (an app that matches mum friends – like Tinder but without the bollocks) campaign to consign phrases like 'incompetent cervix' and 'hostile uterus' to the history books/bin – where they belong!

complex). I really feel that I would have struggled more mentally had I had my children earlier, and that I was 'in the right place' in my life when we had our first son. We must also remember that for many women, having children later is not a choice at all, but something enforced due to circumstances or fertility issues. Waiting, or being forced to wait, can unfortunately equate to some negative physical impacts.

Helen Lauer, a holistic health practitioner, feels this was the case for her: 'I had my daughter at the age of 39. I was an older mum, had a difficult birth, with evident trauma and a significant prolapse visible immediately after the birth. Unfortunately, I did not get signposted to any postpartum care, even with the visible tissue damage. Complications from the grade 4 prolapse, and subsequent hysterectomy some years later, have led to continence issues and a loss of sensation during sex. Being an older mum might have put me at a disadvantage with recovery, but better postpartum care would likely have led to a better outcome for me.' Cyrilynn Preece, a retail manager, was 26 when she had her first child and 39 when she had her twins. Although neither experience was a walk in the park, the first experience was easier as she had a vaginal birth and so was up and about much quicker, and she also felt that she had more support. Her second birth, with the twins, was a c-section and she feels that it was this, and a lack of support, that made recovery harder rather than her age. I also found postpartum mobility easier with my vaginal birth but, other than the mode of birth being different, neither of us found age to be a particularly strong determinant in our recovery.

Indeed, not everyone fares worse for being older. Julie Seal, a creative strategist also known as 'The Chronic Optimist' online, says she feels having a child just before she turned 40 was exactly the right age for her. Julie's story is especially uplifting and reassuring as not only is she an older mum, but she classes herself as part of the 'spoonie' community due to multiple health issues (predominantly the effects of Lyme disease, but with other comorbidities such as POTS*) which had rendered her unable to walk unaided throughout her late 30s. On top of this she is also a solo IVF mother. Yes, you

---

* POTS is an acronym for postural tachycardia syndrome (an abnormal increase in heart rate that occurs after sitting up or standing).

read all of that right. What a mother flipping warrior. Julie told me that she hightailed it down to the fertility clinic as soon as she was told she was in remission from Lyme disease, and her journey into solo motherhood has been 'the most wonderful blessing'. She feels well: the pregnancy hormones have also played a part in dampening down any inflammation or autoimmune 'over-reactions.' Despite a very difficult, traumatic birth which ended with an episiotomy and forceps, she has no lasting physical effects from this. She also adored breastfeeding and did so without any issues, and she has built a strong and supportive community around herself and baby Betsy. Indeed, she feels that parenting can be easier without a partner, 'I genuinely believe it can be easier in many ways. I had had a nightmare husband and I can't think of anything worse than having a baby with a difficult partner. There's also no expectation on anyone else, which they fail to live up to. It's all on me. All the failures and successes are on me and I'm fine with that.' And although it can be lonely at times, Julie has help from her parents and has cultivated a support network that includes other solo mums. In fact, she was gearing up for her first night out on the tiles with them when we spoke. She looked totally at ease and confident in the decision she had made, as daunting as it might be for some people. She said that becoming a mother later on was 'the best thing that has ever happened to me'. Author Genevieve Roberts has written a book called *Going Solo: My choice to become a single mother using a donor* about taking a similar path later in life.

Professor Debra Bick OBE, Professor of Clinical Trials in Maternal Health at Warwick Medical School, adds, 'If older women are planning a first pregnancy, it is really important to stop smoking, limit/stop alcohol intake and think about a healthy diet and maintaining a level of physical activity (walking and swimming for example). There are interventions such as doing pelvic floor muscle exercises, which should be encouraged among all women before and during pregnancy. There is also evidence that perineal massage in a first pregnancy can prevent perineal tears and reduce ongoing perineal pain after the birth.'

## MENOPAUSE

We've discussed menstruation, but what about when that stops, or the years leading up to it (which are called perimenopause)? The postnatal period can mimic some of the same 'symptoms' we feel as we approach menopause and, with women generally older now when starting their families,[65] this can even overlap. I had my second son at 39 and am keeping everything crossed that I have a few years to return to normal, hormonally, and musculoskeletally (perhaps a new term! It's fun to say – try it) before I descend (or ascend, let's put a positive slant on this shizzle) into perimenopause. Women generally start 'becoming menopausal' around age 45, though perimenopause can start much earlier. A recent study[66] has suggested that breastfeeding, particularly extended breastfeeding, can protect against early menopause, with the researchers hypothesising that pregnancies and breastfeeding could lead to later menopause because of 'suppression of ovulation' – this isn't mirrored by taking birth control pills though, and it's not yet clear why. Can you guess what I am going to say next? *More research needed*. Seriously, perhaps I should just write 'more research needed/pending and in the meantime go and see a pelvic health physio… oh and Kegels improve orgasms' and that can be the whole book!

Perimenopause and menopause symptoms can include weight gain, fatigue, low mood, anxiety, joint pain, vaginal dryness, breast tenderness, insomnia, lower sex drive, continence issues, irregular periods, worsening PMS, headaches, brain fog, sweating or hot flushes – much of which you can also experience in the postnatal period as your hormones nose-dive. According to Dr Nighat Arif (a well-known TV doctor), lesser-known symptoms of the menopause can include toothache, a burning tongue, dry mouth, dry skin, and a change in body odour. I'm not going to lie – it does *not* sound a barrel of laughs. Perimenopause and menopause include similar dips in hormone levels, but, unlike postpartum, your hormones won't re-regulate without assistance. Experts such as menopause specialist Dr Louise Newson and former President of the Royal College of Obstetrics and Gynaecology, Dame Lesley Reagan, among others, have worked hard over the years to raise awareness of the challenges of the menopause. I have heard experts say that women are now living for more years in the 'post-fertility' window than in the 'fertile window' and that, while it is wonderful that we have such great life expectancy these days, we are also not designed to live without these hormones (oestrogen, progesterone and testosterone all decrease – among other hormonal changes). All of the experts I spoke to were really keen that women research menopause symptoms and treatments, and speak with health professionals, as hormone replacement therapy and/or lifestyle changes can offer significant improvements in some of the very tricky symptoms and feelings women have during this time. When I spoke to Tracy Allport, an occupational and complementary therapist who now supports women in midlife through a range of different therapies including massage and aromatherapy, she was keen to stress that a holistic approach to the perimenopause and menopause is crucial. Lifestyle factors, such as diet, exercise and stress can really affect how the menopause affects you and 'it is not necessarily as simple as popping a pill (it can take a while to get HRT levels right anyway)'.

One person who promotes an integrated and holistic approach to this next transition phase is consultant gynaecologist and menopause expert, Anne Henderson (www.gynae-expert.co.uk), who has a book called *Natural Menopause*, which aims to help you 'stay physically, mentally, and spiritually well throughout your menopause journey'. I had a chat with her, and was delighted that she could fit me in between clients and the opening of a new women's health clinic in Kent. When we spoke, Anne stressed to me just how much changes in oestrogen levels affect our mind and body function – and that, while women are often aware that the hormone changes can affect their pelvic floor, they are not so well informed about the mental health side-effects. Indeed, Anne has carried out studies in the past about oestrogen levels and postnatal depression. As you can see from the list of symptoms above, both mind and body can be affected by the menopause.

Anne and I chatted about how the postnatal hormone 'crash' can mirror the symptoms of menopause, the difference being that we should 'bounce back' (hormonally) after childbirth and breastfeeding, while perimenopause and menopause create permanent changes. We spoke about what most women did and did not know about menopause. Women may find they now leak urine when they sneeze, laugh or cough, when they didn't before, and they may begin to experience symptoms of pelvic organ prolapse. Anne stated that, while women do tend to know that menopause affects pelvic floor function and continence, they tend to just accept it as 'what would I expect, I am in my fifties and I've had children'. The depletion of oestrogen also affects the tissue of our vaginas, affecting the flexibility and lubrication, which can become uncomfortable and even painful. Oestrogen also affects the lining of the urethra and bladder, helping us to fight off urinary tract infections – so these can increase in frequency when we hit menopause. As with all muscles, we can begin to lose mass as we age and the pelvic floor muscles need to be worked to stay strong, just like any other muscle. If you haven't 'gotten around' to starting pelvic floor exercises, it is never too late. The muscles haven't gone anywhere! They may need reawakening, but they should respond well as you build strength back up. Anne told me that although women do know that their pelvic floor will likely be affected, they don't necessarily bridge the gap between knowledge and action. Action includes making lifestyle changes, building strength and functionality and exploring hormone replacement therapy (HRT).

HRT has had a bad rap due to some inflammatory headlines in the 1990s, which conflated its use with breast cancer and cardiovascular issues. The 'Million Women Study', driven by the University of Oxford,[67] is looking into the long-term effects of menopause hormone therapy, with current findings suggesting that oestrogen-only HRT (and specifically topical, which means applied to the skin) has a low risk profile. Anne also told me that transdermal HRT (patches) is also considered very low risk. There is also oral HRT and something called 'bioidentical hormones'. As with most health issues it's not cut and dried and it's worth exploring what your individual risk profile is, for each type of treatment, and whether the benefits would outweigh the risks. For more information on this, do take a look for the most recent evidence on NHS and government websites. Also, I thought the information on the Cancer Research UK website about HRT was extremely clear and useful.[68]

The MASIC Foundation has worked with Dr Louise Newson on a leaflet* about how taking oestrogen can help with symptoms of birth injuries (including continence and UTI issues). If you have had a bad

---

* https://masic.org.uk/wp-content/uploads/2021/11/Menopause-and-Perineal-Tears-INTERACTIVE.pdf

tear, affecting the anal sphincter muscle, then you may be worried about whether the menopause will affect your bowel control. I've looked at studies, and studies of studies, and it seems that – yes, it might. As tissue and muscles can weaken with age, it follows that the sphincter may be adversely affected – especially if you have sustained any injury during childbirth. And, while you may not experience symptoms as a younger mother, as you age 'there is muscle weakening and changes to the connective tissue which may lengthen, stiffen and/or fail at the time of menopause. It is not until after this point that neural or anal sphincter defects become clinically evident and symptoms of faecal urgency or incontinence develop'.[69] Suffice to say, there needs to be *much more* research in this area, as there is no conclusive evidence as to who will suffer with incontinence, and why, or how best to prevent it. While pelvic floor exercises, and (for some women) hormone replacement therapy, may help prevent symptoms, they are not a panacea. Indeed, one study highlights that, in some women, there was greater reporting of faecal incontinence in those taking oral HRT[70] – although the authors suggest that none of the studies were free from bias and that better quality evidence is sorely needed. So, while it may provide improvements for some women, it is not guaranteed. If you are concerned about this, then do speak to your GP and ask if there is a menopause specialist locally. Also, the MASIC Foundation is a wealth of information and a vital support for anyone suffering with continence issues, or the emotional toll of living with an obstetric injury.

The take-away from all of this is that if, like me, you are potentially going to do a hop, skip and a jump from being postnatal to being perimenopausal then it would serve you well to be prepared. Luckily, the menopause is something that is being increasingly talked about, and better information and support is becoming available. There is now a glut of information out there for you to get your hands on, digest and come up with a plan as to how best to manage this next, potentially tricky, transition. As always, forewarned is forearmed.

## NICU

An area of early motherhood that is seldom discussed, particularly when it comes to postnatal care, is those mothers whose babies have needed neonatal intensive care. I have often had pangs throughout the years as I think about these mothers. I often wondered if they felt even more neglected than the rest of us. My hunch was confirmed when I spoke with two 'NICU mums' – Natalie Dale (featured in case studies in the next chapter for different reasons) and Sam Harrison (www.thenicumummy.co.uk). After traumatic births, both women, who sound like absolute troopers, were left feeling neglected by their lack of postnatal care. After a pretty fraught pregnancy, Sam had an episiotomy and Natalie suffered a bad tear with the birth of her son. Both Sam and Natalie had to cope with additional difficulties in recovery after birth, due to the emotional impact of having a baby in NICU, as well as the added physical demands that being in and out of hospital so much early on can produce. They both struggled with the long walks to and from NICU and to and from the café and/or 'expressing room' and sitting 'bolt upright' on hard chairs.

Sam feels that some people may incorrectly perceive that NICU mums are getting more sleep when at home, when actually either a challenging pumping schedule and/or anxiety about being parted from a poorly baby can both result in extremely poor sleep. Neither Sam nor Natalie had adequate access to midwives or health visitors for postnatal checks and Sam struggled with being denied stronger pain relief because she had been discharged from the labour ward. Some mothers will really struggle with being around other families with newborns and so the postnatal ward, although it gives you access to the medication and medical attention you may need, may be a particularly difficult environment. Natalie and Sam had different experiences with breastfeeding, with Sam able to establish breastfeeding, albeit through an expressing schedule which she felt affected her mental health, and Natalie stopping after a very difficult eight weeks in which a mixture of pumping and breastfeeding did not lead to adequate supply and left Natalie depleted. Both felt that their healing journeys, and breastfeeding, were impacted by the stress of being in NICU. Mothers who want to establish breastfeeding may find it difficult, whether because it is not conducive to the baby's treatment, or because of challenges accessing the right support. Not being able to breastfeed when you want to, particularly when caring for a poorly or vulnerable baby, can trigger extreme feelings – including grief. This is not the place for a diatribe on the treatment of new mothers in NICU, and most parents stress their extreme gratitude to the NICU staff for how well they have looked after their vulnerable babies (often going above and beyond), but suffice to say hospital policies and culture need to be looked at to ensure these women are being properly cared for as well – and that proper funding is available to ensure it is actually feasible!

Sam spends a lot of time raising awareness about the plight of NICU parents, and runs a very active website, with a blog, and Instagram and Twitter accounts. She fosters an understanding community for others going through the same, or similar, ordeals. Sam and Natalie gave me some excellent advice to pass on to new mothers who find themselves in NICU:

- Ask for a side room if you are on or near the postnatal ward, so that you are not surrounded by newborns.
- Take in your own pregnancy pillow or similar, and maybe a doughnut ring pillow, to try and make yourself more comfortable.
- Don't worry about asking the staff for things for yourself (such as seeing a breastfeeding specialist, or if they could let you know about the meal trolley and doctors rounds). You are not being a nuisance, you matter too.
- If aiming to breastfeed, ask doctors, nurses, and midwives to co-produce a plan with you to avoid conflicting information and advice. Also ask if you can pump next to your baby as this may help with milk release, and ease anxiety about being parted from your baby. See if your partner, if you have one, can help by sterilising and labelling bottles.
- Conversely, if you are feeling pressurised to breastfeed and it's not working for you, you can also ask the hospital if they have breastfeeding targets to reach. You do not need to be a statistic.
- Ask hospital staff if they have a reclining chair so you can nap during the day.
- Ask staff for a permit for the carpark so you don't have to pay for parking.
- If you have an older child, take in a photo to put on the little cupboard they give you.

- Take earplugs and/or headphones to enable you to tune out the other noises and allow you to nap.
- Have a very large water bottle (so you don't have to make too many trips to the kitchen).
- Take slippers/warm socks for wards and flip-flops for the toilet/bathroom area, especially if you attempt to use the shower.
- Accept any offers of help from friends and family.

Sam points out that it can feel odd accepting help if you haven't brought your baby home with you, but that you are just as deserving, if not more so, of support. If friends and family are not sure how they can help, you can suggest that they make healthy food boxes up that you can take into hospital with you or heat up at home once you get back. Microwavable dishes of home-cooked food will always be appreciated, and if it's ready-labelled with your name then it will make life a little easier. Equally, any healthy cold snacks they can make or deliver to you, to keep you going when you are at the baby's bedside, will be welcome.

I would add to the above that if you have not received a proper check postnatally, that your partner, friend or parent requests this for you.

Finally, Sam makes the particularly important point *not to put yourself last*. It is natural to focus all of your energy on your baby, whether they go home healthy with you or have to spend time in NICU. Obviously being in NICU will likely stir up all sorts of difficult and challenging emotions, as well as you feeling exhausted and potentially very sore from the birth. To be the mum you want to be, it's important to ensure you recharge when you can and get any of your own health issues addressed too. You will not be able to be as present as you'd like to be if you suffer any post-birth complication, so note any aches, pains, fevers, strange-smelling discharge or anything that feels 'not quite right' and insist on being seen. If it is too upsetting to be seen on the postnatal ward, and I wholeheartedly agree that this would be traumatic, then you can strongly request to be seen on a different ward or in a side-room. As I've said repeatedly, you need to be an advocate for yourself and your own health. It might feel like a step too far at the moment, but it will pay dividends later if you can get any physical issues seen to promptly.

I am not going to harp on too much about things you should/ shouldn't be doing during this very difficult period, but I will give you one thing to think about *trying* to do if you can muster the energy. Breathing properly will help reduce your stress levels and gently work your pelvic floor and abdominal muscles. As your pelvic floor works in 'partnership' with your diaphragm, it is important to release tension from this area. Deep breaths (feeling the breath go right out into your side ribs, with a little going to your belly) and long, slow out-breaths will help release tension and the exhale also helps 'lift' the pelvic floor. If you can start thinking about a 'jelly fish' motion around your pelvic area as you breathe in and out, this might help give the pelvic floor a little workout and encourage blood flow to the pelvic area, which will help with healing. Another little trick is the 'timed breath' – breathing in for a count of four, and out for a count of six. According to neuroscientist Professor Ian Robertson, controlling your breath in this way 'can change your heart rate, lower your blood pressure, reduce your stress levels and combat anxiety, reduce feelings of pain and even change your brain chemistry to make your mind sharper.'[71] And if there's anywhere that you need this technique, I'd say NICU is the place. One thing that many of you might not think of, likely because you will not have heard of it, is 'binding' or 'wrapping' your abdomen. Doula Sophie Messager suggests wrapping your abdomen – especially if you've had a c-section – 'as this may help you move more easily'. She talks at length about this traditional practice in her book *Why Postnatal Recovery Matters*.

Talking about your experience might be a good way of dealing with the stress, anxiety and upset – or, indeed, the trauma. It might be best to start working through these emotions sooner rather than later, with someone you trust and feel comfortable with. More resources are at the back of the book.

## MISCARRIAGE AND STILLBIRTH/NEONATAL DEATH

If there has been a feeling that no one really talks about your postnatal body, or cares about it, I felt that triple-fold after suffering with recurrent miscarriage. Obviously, the emotional toll was huge, but it doesn't exist on its own. Your body is still making major adjustments, and that is very rarely recognised or discussed. The NHS website briefly mentions how breastmilk continues to be produced after a stillbirth or neonatal death, but there is scant information on your postpartum body after loss.

Pregnancy loss and stillbirth are difficult and hugely emotive subjects to tackle. I even wondered whether to include this section in the book, as I know I found it scary to see these terms anywhere when I was pregnant. But the reality is that at least one in four of us will experience pregnancy loss and, although stillbirth and neonatal death are much less common, they do still happen. No one wants to think about it, and my goodness, I don't blame you. So, feel free to skip this part, but for those of you who have experienced this heart-wrenching loss – this is for you.

***Pregnancy loss and your body.*** My first miscarriage was a 'missed miscarriage' (can I take a second to say I hate this term for its double blame-laden undertone. Feeling that I had 'missed' the fact that I had 'miscarried' – a term I find thoughtless and old-fashioned – was an extra paper cut of words that I could have done without) at almost 12 weeks, and it was absolutely not what I had heard about or was expecting. Without going in to too much detail, as it is a long and pretty gruesome tale, I was in and out of A&E and experienced extremely heavy blood loss, cramps that were reminiscent of labour pains, vomiting and a fever. I was on a drip twice and was pretty close to also needing a blood transfusion. Some people assume miscarriages are like heavy periods, and indeed, my third miscarriage was like that as it was much earlier on (about six weeks), but everyone is different. How many weeks gone you are will likely have an impact on how you are *physically* affected, but the emotional toll, at any point during gestation, can be huge and suffice to say that all feelings are valid. Your anguish might be just as overwhelming at the very beginning of a pregnancy as it is later on. For more help and support on the emotional side of things, please take a look at Tommy's website and resources. I am sorry for your loss, I am sorry you are experiencing this – it is so very, very hard.

With missed miscarriages, you may have the ordeal of carrying the baby until your body decides to begin the process of miscarrying or until you can get booked in for medical/surgical management. I know how hard this is. Just do what works for you to get through this. To be simultaneously pregnant, and not pregnant, is an awful feeling. For me to get through it, I wore huge jumpers and did distracting things like taking my older son to the woods. For you it may be cradling your tummy and saying goodbye. Everything is valid, there is no right or wrong way to deal with this awful situation.

After a pregnancy loss, you may feel weak due to the blood loss, and your abdomen may be tender – particularly if you have had to have a surgical procedure to help clear your womb. This used to be an ERPC (evacuation of retained products of conception) but is mostly now referred to as SMM (surgical management of miscarriage). I am sorry if, like me, you find these terms quite distressing to hear/read. I have experienced both 'natural' miscarriages and SMM and both have needed a significant chunk of recovery time. After your pregnancy loss, you will likely need to be checked by ultrasound to assess whether your womb is clear of 'pregnancy tissue' (more clunky terminology) which is what you might like to think of as 'your baby', to ensure you have a decreased risk of infection in your womb. This test will involve a probe being inserted into your vagina as this is the easiest way to get a clear picture of your womb. You may have already been through this at a scan when you were still pregnant, and it may feel traumatic and intrusive as a result. It's not pleasant but it shouldn't be uncomfortable, and the sonographer should be gentle and sensitive. It can feel a lot to contend with after a loss, but try to do your deep breathing so that your muscles relax and try to keep your jaw loose (I know how tempting it is to literally grit your teeth as you think 'just get through this next bit'). Remember an 'in breath' is what actually enables your pelvic floor to relax. You will also likely have a series of follow-up blood tests to check your iron levels. You may need to take iron and B12 supplements to help restore your levels and also help give you more energy. I experienced pretty extreme fatigue after my first miscarriage, which lasted for weeks, and my blood loss was such that I could not sit up without feeling light-headed and like I could hear crashing waves and a clock chiming (which my scientist husband explained to me was low blood pressure). The only cure for this was rest, getting enough fluids and supplements.

You may find that you also have your hCG (human chorionic gonadotropin) levels checked. This is a hormone involved in the development of the placenta, which indicates pregnancy. The reason for this is that during and after a miscarriage, hCG levels should drop. If they don't, it could be that you are experiencing an ectopic pregnancy (where a fertilised egg implants outside the womb – usually in a fallopian tube) and this will mean you need urgent medical attention. Rising hCG levels are one of the culprits for pregnancy nausea or 'morning sickness', as well as breast tenderness, so when these drop you may be relieved of these symptoms. I am well aware that these symptoms disappearing can be anything but a relief. Pregnancy symptoms disappearing is absolutely not always a sign of any issue or pregnancy loss, but when they do go hand in hand it can be very hard to deal with and you may end up missing the very symptoms you were cursing only days earlier. This is normal. As well as hCG levels subsiding, your oestrogen and progesterone levels will also drop, which can intensify your feelings of trauma and loss. Eventually they will return to pre-pregnancy levels, though I have struggled to find much research on the timeframe for this – it is thought to be a matter of weeks rather than months.

If you have had surgical management of miscarriage, you will almost certainly have had a general anaesthetic, which can make you feel nauseous, fatigued, achy or dizzy – among other, less common, side-effects. You may also find you have disturbed sleep after general anaesthetic,[72] which is unhelpful for recovery and your general psychological state. I found it best not to try and strive for sleep and I actually went downstairs and video-called a friend in Australia as I knew she would be up. This was the best course of action for me at the time, but to enable your body to recover, using a meditation or sleep hypnosis track may feel more beneficial.

When I spoke with Jennie Agg, a journalist who has written extensively, and extremely insightfully, about her own experience of recurrent miscarriage, she also cited insomnia as a postpartum symptom after miscarriage. Jennie endured four losses before the birth of her son, Edward, and each time she suffered with the type of insomnia that she now recognises as 'pregnancy insomnia' as it was a very similar feeling to the later stages of her last pregnancy. She told me that she experienced this insomnia after her losses whether she had had general anaesthesia or not. We spoke about the dearth of research into women's postpartum bodies after pregnancy loss and how we don't know how much the fatigue, insomnia and also joint instability (Jennie went running soon after her first miscarriage in a bid to feel normal again and felt vulnerable to injury) is related to grief, and how much to hormones. It seems that the narrative around miscarriages being common has meant that they are construed as 'normal' and also 'no big thing', which means that women can struggle with recovery and being given the time to recover properly. Indeed, Jennie felt that she approached her 'recovery' in a way that was detrimental to her physical and mental health after her first miscarriage. Numbed by grief, but within a system and society that does not yet fully recognise the intensity of this grief, she pushed herself to not only 'carry on as normal', but also to drive her body too far, too fast. Reflecting, she said that perhaps she was angry with her body and the way she channelled this was to work harder, run faster and try to get pregnant again as quickly as possible, as she didn't want to be hanging around waiting. This went against the gentle advice she had been given by a colleague who had been through it herself – to 'rest, relax and take her time'. In hindsight, Jennie says she wishes she had adopted this approach and been kinder to herself and her body.

After the pain and fatigue have calmed down, you may still experience bleeding for a number of days or weeks – depending how far along you were. You must monitor this discharge for anything that could indicate that the pregnancy loss has left tissue in your womb or there is infection. Things to look out for include blood loss worsening and soaking through more than one pad an hour, any odd smell, or blood loss continuing longer than your healthcare provider has indicated. Also, any acute or lingering abdominal pain, shoulder tip pain and/or a fever should be investigated. You may also have tender breasts for a while and a rounded tummy. In fact, I found I looked more pregnant between my miscarriages than after the birth of my second son. I wonder if this is partly because I felt vulnerable about that area and was not working on core strength at all – coupled with a wodge of comfort eating – as well as the up and down hormonal shifts of being pregnant/not pregnant/pregnant again and so on.

Both Jennie and my friend, Claire, also noticed that their tummies stayed rounded after their miscarriages – even if the losses were fairly early on. Jennie told me she lived in fear of someone wondering, or even asking, if she was pregnant and said it felt particularly cruel to look pregnant after loss. I completely agree. I felt very disconnected from my tummy and womb when I was experiencing recurrent miscarriage. I didn't really touch or look at my abdomen and I hid my body in very baggy clothes and felt unable to connect enough to do the Pilates or yoga that I loved so much beforehand. I also let my pelvic floor exercises slide. I guess I felt angry at my body too. I have realised now that what my body really needed was nurturing. I had some counselling, which I mainly used as a chance to release some emotion and frustration, but I found complementary therapies such as reiki, fertility massage and acupuncture really helped me reconnect with my body. Having someone else touch my abdomen in such a nurturing way, when I was unable to myself, was so very healing.

A post-pregnancy bump, and breasts that might still be heavier – or even leaking – can be a painful reminder of what you have lost. To help with breast discomfort, or leaking, you can gently massage your breasts in the shower. If this is too upsetting, you can ask your healthcare provider or GP if they would prescribe a dopamine-agoniser drug to suppress lactation. A recent framework for lactation after stillbirth[73] states that 'We would also caution against brief ambiguous statements that can sometimes accompany information endorsing gentle suppression. Specificity in how to gently suppress milk supply, without making more milk, is likely to be required by parents who may have little lactation experience and may not know how to confidently express for the purpose of suppression'. Essentially, the authors worry that a mother being told to go away and manually pump to relieve pressure and discomfort may either do too much (and therefore increase supply rather than decrease it) or too little – putting her at risk of mastitis and breast abscesses. If you opt for 'gentle suppression' by massaging/pumping, then do keep an eye out for any red patches, rashes, or bumps on the breasts, and acute or dull pain and any fever – as these can be signs of mastitis which would likely need a course of antibiotics.

My most surprising physical after-effect of miscarriage was hair loss. It wasn't as extreme as my full-term postpartum hair loss, but it was still something I hadn't been expecting. I hadn't even realised I'd stopped shedding hair when I showered, so to be pulling out quite large clumps when washing my hair was an unpleasant revelation and added an extra layer of sadness, as just another reminder of what might've been.

**Stillbirth and neonatal death.** Your body may be the last thing on your mind after experiencing stillbirth or losing your baby after birth (neonatal death). Unfortunately, our bodies will still behave as they would if you had been able to take your baby home. This can come as a crushing shock and be deeply distressing.

As I have not experienced late pregnancy loss/baby loss, stillbirth or neonatal death, I asked mothers who had experienced this if they would feel comfortable sharing with me their postpartum experience. I was overwhelmed with the generosity of these women, who, having already been through so much, were willing to reflect on this difficult time and share their experiences to help others.

Alex Barr, a staff nurse from Dorset, lost her daughter, Marnie, in 2020, which has been proven to have been due to clinical negligence. She told me 'There really is no mention of your postnatal body after loss of any kind, that I'm aware of, and in my case stillbirth. While in hospital and then when home, no healthcare professional had any kind of discussion about how I was feeling physically.' She went on to explain how the emptiness felt truly physical, as well as emotional, and that she now knows she suffered with 'empty arms syndrome', which manifested as a real ache in her arms, such was her need to hold her baby. Alex's grief had a massive impact on her recovery. 'It impacted my ability to think clearly and to be able to look after myself. Initially, I had no desire to eat, drink, take painkillers to help with the discomfort of endometritis (a womb infection caused by the birth), exercise or sleep.' Alex already had an older son so she was aware that she should have had a postnatal check-up, and she knew how important all of the above was for her healing, but she was understandably struggling so much emotionally that it took all of her will just to get out of bed every day, for the sake of her family. She found her family a huge support in encouraging her to do little things each day, such as cooking from scratch together to both distract and nourish her, but she found it extremely hard that she was abandoned by her healthcare providers. 'It was as if my postnatal health didn't matter because my baby had died.'

Alex took cabergoline (a stimulant of dopamine receptors in the brain which also inhibits release of prolactin by the pituitary) to stop her lactating, but she still experienced some symptoms, which she found very difficult to deal with. She had not contemplated her milk coming in and she took the medication to help relieve some of this added trauma. Alex also did regular sitz baths, once her womb infection had cleared, with lavender and witch hazel to help treat her small tear, as 'your grief is even worse when you are physically in pain from giving birth. In my experience, this pain is much easier to deal with when you have a baby in your arms, not when they are empty.' On that note, Alex recommends two ways to help ease the 'empty arms syndrome' she suffered: first, taking the time to really hug any children you may already have, and second, connecting with Aching Arms – a charity founded by bereaved parents who provide comfort teddy bears for other parents to hold on to as they go through the grieving process. Alex describes grief as 'not linear, it's messy and unkind and it has a massive impact on you physically.' She went on to have another child via caesarean section which she felt helped her in the postpartum period as it was not reminiscent of her other birthing experiences and gave her an element of control. For other mothers going through this awful experience, Alex recommends taking each day as it comes, sleeping when you feel tired, eating wholesome food and exercising when you can: 'Home-cooked, fresh, healthy foods really helped the physical recovery. We also did a lot of walking too, to try and get out and make sense of what had happened. Although this felt like the biggest hurdle each time, just to leave the house, when we did – it really did help.'

I also spoke with a local friend, Lucy Bennington, about her experience after losing her daughter, Amber. Amber passed away at nine days old after being treated in NICU for severe hypoxia (lack of oxygen). Lucy is keen to stress that many babies with hypoxia make a full recovery, but they were not so lucky. She told me how physical the pain is after such a seismic loss. She told me she was floored by how her arms physically ached and how her chest hurt as if she could feel her heart breaking. Lucy was given Sudafed to help reduce milk production, which is an 'off-label' use (i.e. where the clinical studies to demonstrate the treatment is effective for that indication have not yet been done), which she felt worked, and some steroids for the hives which covered her stomach and legs.

It was illuminating speaking to Lucy, as it was so obvious that the emotions, and the physical manifestation of these emotions, were so clear she could almost touch them, but any physical discomfort was much harder to recall. This was despite an episiotomy, forceps delivery, losing a lot of blood and being so weak she almost passed out. This goes to show how little attention women going through this trauma are able to pay to their bodies, and how much care from others they therefore need. After saying goodbye to Amber, Lucy knew she really needed the care of her own parents. Luckily, both her parents and her partner's stepped in. Lucy says, 'Dave went home and cleared all the baby stuff away. I went back to my parents, and just stayed. There was never a conversation, it just happened.' Lucy says this period of time with her parents was what really helped her heal, more so than any subsequent therapy. This is because her parents not only cossetted her, but allowed her to replay the events again and again as she tried to make sense of what had happened. She felt she could also break down emotionally as much as she needed. This was reflected back to her by her parents, who, having also been present at the birth, were suffering immense anguish as well. Lucy says that this way of grieving freely, and together, and the permission to relive the experience, was healing. She also remembers sitting with her mum brushing her hair, as she felt too weak to do anything for herself. Her mum felt the need to mother her daughter in this way, and Lucy felt that she needed it. Lucy also tells me that she found taking baths very therapeutic, as being in the water itself felt healing, and she feels it encourages the tears out. Lucy went on to have two sons after Amber, Nathan and Rupert, and she chose planned caesarean sections, the same as Alex. She felt very well-cared for throughout her pregnancies, although they were anxious times. She was surprised at how fast she healed after the abdominal births, although the second one was tougher as she already had a high-energy three-year-old to look after. Lucy feels her care after losing Amber was poor, with a lack of empathy from some staff in the hospital as well as her GP at the six-week check. Lucy's advice, for anyone in a similarly heartbreaking situation, is to reach out to other mothers going through it too. She said, 'It's the club no one wants to join, but they are the only ones who will understand. You form such a strong bond with these other women. I am still in touch, years later. We get each other through it.'

You may also have to deal with many of the things we've already discussed, but without having your baby beside you. This may make the symptoms harder to deal with, and where I was light-hearted in tone in earlier chapters, this is unlikely to resonate with you. So below, I summarise the most common immediate postpartum 'symptoms':

**Lochia** – you will experience bleeding from your vagina, whether you had a vaginal or caesarean birth, for weeks after the birth. If the blood loss increases in volume, with large clots, or you notice an unpleasant smell, you should flag this to your healthcare provider. Use maternity pads or heavy-duty sanitary pads rather than tampons or menstrual cups and change them regularly to prevent infection.

**Blood loss** – if you have lost a lot of blood, you may need to keep an eye on your iron and B12 levels. Taking a gentle supplement will not harm you if you can't face more tests and may help with the fatigue that both birth and grief can cause.

**Breasts** – you may experience breast engorgement as your breasts fill with milk. This can make your breasts feel heavy, tender and the skin may feel tight. You can massage your breasts gently to release the milk (in a warm shower might be easiest) and use a gentle pulling motion around the areola (you can put a thumb underneath and your other fingers on top, about an inch up from your areola and squeeze and draw downwards slightly). Try to just relieve the pain and discomfort, as if you fully empty each breast then it can signal to your body to produce *more* milk rather than to slow down milk production. You can opt to donate your breastmilk, if you feel this would help you come to terms with what has happened, and you can get more information and support at The Human Milk Foundation (www.humanmilkfoundation. org). Alternatively, you can ask your healthcare provider for drugs to stop lactation, as many women will find producing milk incredibly distressing after losing a baby.

**Vagina** – giving birth can be very taxing on your vagina and you may be swollen and sore. You may have stitches from tearing or an episiotomy. To help heal your stitches, try to shower regularly, and lie down to let the area air-dry. Make sure your midwife, GP or health visitor checks your stitches to ensure you are healing, and if there is any odd coloured or smelly discharge then flag it with them, as it can be a sign of infection. Your vagina should start feeling less sore within 1–2 weeks and if it isn't, then do speak to someone about this. Alex Barr, who spoke to me about her experience of stillbirth, recommended regular sitz baths to help your stitches heal. Although it will probably seem like the last thing to be concerned about, your body will thank you if you start doing your pelvic floor exercises early on. Just gentle breathing out as you pull up your muscles (as if you are stopping wee mid-flow and stopping passing wind at the same time) and breathing in as you fully release and relax a few times throughout the day (and then build on these, using something like the Squeezy app, as you begin to feel stronger) will be an investment in your future health and continence. It may be very tempting to ignore this part of your body – your tummy, womb, and pelvic floor. I can relate to that. Don't put pressure on yourself, but it might be worth consciously trying to engage with this area as disconnecting can be detrimental to your long-term health. You may need assistance to help you do this – whether through bereavement or other psychological counselling, or more body-based therapy such as reiki, massage, acupuncture or even specialist womb massage – but reconnecting and nourishing your abdomen and pelvis and focusing on regaining strength in this area will help you to reap benefits not just for future pregnancies and births, but also for sustaining quality of life as you get older.

**Your bum** – piles and constipation. These two go hand-in-hand and nobody wants either. Constipation is truly the enemy of a decent postnatal recovery and may likely be a familiar foe from pregnancy.

As your nutrition and hydration may take a real battering due to the trauma you have experienced, constipation (or, conversely, diarrhoea) may be a daily blight. Grieving people are particularly at risk of dehydration and I will repeat my constant refrain: *hydrate*. I really hope someone is looking after you and keeping you watered and well fed. But if you are shouldering looking after yourself after this awful loss, please, if you do nothing else – eat little and often (I am not going to preach about nutrition) and make sure you have enough to drink (about 1.5–2 litres per day in water, juices, and teas). Blood clots are more common after giving birth and being dehydrated can add to that risk.

Piles (haemorrhoids) can make sitting down and going to the toilet extremely uncomfortable after birth. Rest assured they should reduce and calm down within days or weeks and keeping bowel habits regular will help eliminate constipation – which is the main cause of piles. As well as avoiding constipation, sitz baths may also help with this and you can get over-the-counter creams from any pharmacy and online from supermarkets too.

You may find other parts of this book helpful during your physical recovery, but equally there may be too many mentions of babies and it might be too triggering for you. In that instance, try reaching out to your hospital to see if you can have access to the bereavement midwife (all hospital Trusts should have one) or check out Tommy's charity, which enables you to access advice and support from midwives.

## A WORD ON GRIEF

Grief physically impacts the body. Whether you have been through miscarriage, stillbirth, or neonatal death you will likely experience feelings of grief. There is a huge spectrum of grief, as there is with any other emotion. Marie Curie (the cancer support charity) lists some of the most common physical ailments or feelings you may experience if you are grieving:

- a hollow feeling in your stomach
- tightness in your chest or throat
- oversensitivity to noise
- difficulty breathing

- feeling very tired and weak
- a lack of energy
- dry mouth
- an increase or decrease in appetite
- finding it hard to sleep or fear of sleeping
- aches and pains

In addition, grief can adversely affect your immune system and blood pressure, so, as difficult as it is, it is essential that you try to maintain or establish some healthy habits as you recover from the birth and loss. The bereavement charity Cruse suggests that you keep a food diary if you experience digestion difficulties, and eat smaller portions of healthy food if you can. They also recommend that you keep to a regular bedtime and find time to rest in the day if you are struggling with sleep, and also maintain some sort of exercise such as walking in nature. I recommend finding ways to boost your immune system, through diet or supplements, as dealing with minor illnesses on top of grief will add more of a burden to your body – and your mind. Something as simple as remembering to take a daily high-quality multi-vitamin might make a significant difference. Tommy's, Sands and Bliss charities all have great advice online about how to come to terms with what happened to you, including a note from Tommy's to try not to 'numb' the pain with alcohol, as you will likely feel worse once the effects wear off.

The body and mind are linked and should be treated as such. Being able to express yourself, in whatever way works for you, whether that be talking with friends and family, finding other parents who have gone through the same thing, journaling or talking with a counsellor who specialises in bereavement, will likely help you work through some of your emotions. I recall an acupuncturist I visited when I was going through the miscarriages telling me that if I pushed my feelings down, instead of letting them out, they would find another way out of me. I was often run down in this period, and I think she was right about my grief manifesting itself within my body. I am not sure that I did talk about what I was going through enough, although I did try counselling. With hindsight, had I addressed my emotions more thoroughly and been more open, I might have felt more comfortable and well in my body.

In her book *Why Postnatal Recovery Matters*, doula Sophie Messager advocates for the use of a 'closing the bones' ceremony (a traditional postpartum practice, in which a trained birthworker will wrap and rock your pelvis and abdomen). I can certainly see how some women would find this healing and it puts a focus on your emotional and physical recovery.

Exercise may seem like a step too far, but having a walk in the fresh air, or doing some movement (such as yoga) which feels nurturing to your body, could help a little. It won't take away your pain, but it will help your body feel better equipped to carry you through this difficult time. I have mentioned Bettina Rae already. She produces online yoga sessions which cover recovery after pregnancy loss, and I found these incredibly gentle and helpful. I believe that emotions do need to work their way through your body, and yoga – coupled with good breathing techniques – can really help facilitate this. In addition, after loss, and where that loss has happened within us, or with a part of us, it can be tempting to shut off from or punish your body. If you can, use the yoga principle of practising non-violence towards yourself and your body by treating it kindly. Imagine if what had happened to you had happened to a friend. How would you treat them? Try to apply that feeling to your body. You live in your body forever, so making peace with it, treating it as you would a friend, showing it respect, gently leading it through the grief and the healing, will only have a positive impact on you.

## MENTAL HEALTH ISSUES

You are reading this book because you want to increase your knowledge about what happens to your body postnatally. However, the mind and the body are not separate, and one intrinsically affects the other. A 2000 study[74] highlighted how much more common depression was in mothers who were experiencing postpartum physical complaints such as incontinence, perineal and back pain, and dyspareunia (pain during sex) – as well as fatigue and feeling run down. We should not underestimate how our physical health impacts our mood. Another, more recent study[75] concludes that 'poor physical health in the early postnatal period is associated with poorer mental health throughout the first 12 months postpartum'. I'm glad these studies have been done, but I'd also say it's hardly rocket science that if you are physically depleted, exhausted and in pain, that you may not feel like a ray of ruddy sunshine! It is also worth noting that alongside the huge change to your way of life and possibly your identity, you have also undergone the largest hormonal shift you will ever experience and 'mental disturbances due to hormonal changes following childbirth have been mentioned in medical literature since Hippocrates'.[76]

However, mood disorders are complex and are rooted in a variety of different causes. Postnatal mood 'disorders' are incredibly common, with around 1 in 10 women experiencing postnatal depression and/ or postnatal anxiety and 1 in 25 women experiencing PTSD (post-traumatic stress disorder) symptoms. These mood disorders are something very different, and much longer-lasting, than the 'baby blues,' which is a common (if not universal) mood dip that happens a few days after the birth and coincides with plummeting oestrogen and progesterone levels. The baby blues can leave you feeling very teary and overwhelmed, but should only last a few days.

Postnatal depression is often characterised by a persistent low mood, sleep disturbances (even when baby is sleeping), feeling hopeless and guilty. Postnatal anxiety may be characterised by feeling unable to relax, being irritable, experiencing racing thoughts or even panic attacks. Less common are PTSD (where you might get flashbacks to the birth, feel out of control, or have intrusive thoughts about dying, or are 'hyper-vigilant' around the baby) and postnatal psychosis, whereby you might experience very extreme mood swings, intrusive thoughts, hallucinations, and confusion. If this all sounds scary, rest assured there is much more understanding of, and support for, postnatal mental health issues than there used to be. Women with mental health issues are often swiftly put on a care pathway which will lead them to a full recovery.

Over on social media, and in print, more and more women are talking about maternal 'rage', from writer Saima Mir in *The Best Most Awful Job* to Dr Caroline Boyd on Instagram. While maternal rage is something that may surface later on in motherhood, as expectation and reality clash and the weight of the mental load takes its toll, it can also be a sign of postnatal depression. If any of the above sounds like you, do flag it to your GP and also take a look at PANDAS organisation (details at the back of the book).

Even if you are not in a position where you would be diagnosed with a mental health issue, most of the questions asked about your mental health (usually on a questionnaire) in the postpartum period may resonate with you. Feeling sleep-deprived, exhausted, irritable, tearful, anxious, and hopeless *can* be part of your every day in the early transition into motherhood. Also, mood disorders may surface later on in your postnatal journey – not just at the beginning. Cumulative sleep disturbances, environmental and relationship factors/issues, slow physical healing, and hormonal shifts can all play their part in your mental health. For some mothers, the return of their periods, or weaning their baby off breastmilk, can signal some disruptions to their mood. Dr Emma Svanberg, a clinical psychologist with a specialism in helping mothers, and mothers-to-be, has raised awareness of these less-often talked about aspects of motherhood and how hormonal transitions can impact on our mental health. Emma is a strong advocate for trying talking therapies before or alongside medication (if appropriate). If you are ready to wean, try to do it gradually, as sudden changes in hormones could lead to a real drop in mood, and ask someone to help you monitor whether this is having an impact (often others spot these changes in us before we do).

I spoke to Emma about how we can try to recover mind, body, and soul after pregnancy and birth. It was an insightful chat, in which we both lamented the pressure society places on mothers to return to the body, life and career they had pre-baby, but without giving us the structure and support to do that – and without questioning whether that is where we should be headed anyway. Emma, in her lovely lilting north-east tones, impressed on me how unrealistic and how unfair the expectations we set on new mothers are, and how detrimental this is to their full recovery after birth. Emma said that it consistently 'blew her mind' how women were expected to cope with newborn babies, and sometimes older children, after c-sections and difficult births, with little to no support. How what is essentially a massive feat of endurance day after day is minimised and leaves women feeling like they are not coping as 'other women do this every day'. On top of that, our ordinary 'coping strategies' which enable us to stay on top of our mental health (such as running, or having time alone) have vanished overnight, which can leave us floundering.

Emma talked about the lack of role models who show the reality of postpartum bodies and lives, and how this affects where we think we should be. When I asked Emma about how women could get back to the 'highs' they normally get from high-impact activity or career successes, when we are asking them to go slower to help their postpartum recovery, Emma framed it as a chance to step back and look objectively at our lives and what is being expected of us. She referenced Dr Rangan Chatterjee[77] and his focus on how modern living creates stress in our lives. Early parenthood, and the sleep deprivation that comes with it, raises our cortisol anyway, so on top of our modern 'productivity and high adrenalin' focused model of living, we can find ourselves thoroughly overworked. Emma feels this period of time, especially in 'the fourth trimester', when we can effectively 'step out of society and off that treadmill', could be a time to refocus on what our bodies need, and what pace we are actually comfortable at. This approach really resonated with me. I absolutely feel we are catapulted 'back into the real world' too fast after such a huge physical undertaking and monumental life change. Taking the time to readjust our focus, tune in to our bodies and find what serves us best 'now,' at this new time, where you can slow down and get in step with your baby, is well worth considering. In all likelihood, life will be back to the high-octane pace we are used to in a shorter amount of time than you imagine, so why not try and embrace this pause? Going slowly will feel alien, and may be a really hard adaptation in itself, but giving yourself the permission to do so (where it does not, generally, come from our society as a whole) may feel like a wonderful act of liberation, and the kindest thing you can do for your body. And what is good for the body, is also good for the mind and the soul.

Emma and I spoke about how your mental health can affect your physical recovery post-birth, and vice versa. Emma was clear that, if a woman speaks about some mental health difficulties after the birth, and these are minimised, then she may not feel confident to bring up physical complaints, which can lead to undiagnosed postnatal issues (including undiagnosed severe tears). Equally, if a woman's physical experience or issues are minimised, she may not feel able to broach any mental health issues she may be encountering. During research for my campaign, and this book, this is something I came across time and time again. It shook me how often the dismissal of women's pain and physical challenges postpartum led to an alarming and severe downward spiral. It can be so hard to speak up in those early days, so having an advocate (a partner, doula, sibling, mother, friend) to help you express yourself and be understood, can be so very helpful.

With regards to the mental and physical interplay in the postpartum period, we spoke about how fragmented care can be and how a holistic model would be so much more beneficial – given the myriad of emotions and mental and physical health issues that pregnancy and birth can throw up. As Emma says, she is a clinical psychologist, and she is not trained in manual trauma release or hormones and these things can have huge impacts on mental health. Luckily, she says, there is a shift in direction to a more holistic approach, with people like her colleague – Dr Becca Moore – pioneering treatment in this area. So, if you have a referral or prescription, or are pursuing one area of treatment – do look into what other therapies or specialists *might* be able to help you as well.

I asked Emma how women could become more accepting of their postpartum bodies, given the extensive criticism I have seen women levelling at themselves throughout my research for this book. Emma says that part of the issue is unrealistic expectations, which are bred early. We are taught from an early age that our worth is tied into our appearance, and this is deeply embedded in our society. It is also what allows 'diet culture' to thrive, whereby an industry makes billions of pounds feeding off insecurities it helped to create. But beyond that, and beyond the 'body positivity' movement, which may not quite fit with how a woman feels after birth, there is 'the compassionate approach'. She says, 'Recognising what your body has been through and honouring that and, also, looking at it from a place of kindness. If you are working against your body, punishing it, or feeling disconnected from it, this is not a good foundation for balance or good physical and mental health. If the birth was difficult, or you had a hard pregnancy, or difficulty becoming pregnant, you could feel at odds with your body. So, using this time to reconnect and show compassion will help foster a better long-term relationship with your body'. You might as well make friends with your body – it's not going anywhere! Seriously, you have to live in your body your whole life, so showing it kindness (rubbing a cream or oil into your parched skin, going for a massage or pedicure) will provoke good feelings and also lower your stress levels. With regards to fitness, Emma thinks classes with a focus on compassion toward your body and building strength, rather than focusing too heavily on aesthetics, are the way forward, citing classes like yoga and Pilates.

Help is widely available now if you are experiencing distressing mental health issues postpartum. These can sometimes be more difficult to access if you come from a marginalised community, for a variety of reasons, and in those instances, charities can be incredibly helpful at helping to guide you or help you advocate for yourself. These are listed at the back of the book. Not all practitioners are created equal. So, if you are referred for a talking therapy, and the relationship is not working for you – do try another therapist. Equally, it is worth checking out some of the 'complementary' therapies in Chapter 9 as it may take more than one type of therapy to help you heal.

# CHAPTER 8

# REAL-LIFE INSIGHTS, CASE STUDIES AND ADVICE FROM OTHER MUMS

If I was the reader, rather than the writer, of this book, I would flip to this section first. This is because, for all the stats and information from experts, *this* is where I'd go to see if I was 'normal'. The raw, real, relatable information you get from your peers is kind of unsurpassable when it comes to making you feel more normal, whatever you are experiencing. That is why forums (whether for mothers or for those living with health conditions) are so popular and rife with threads about symptoms and the diagnosing/ management thereof. When I spoke to journalist Jennie Agg about women's bodies after pregnancy loss, she spoke about a few of the phenomena that seem to be commonly experienced. These included insomnia, joint instability, stubborn weight gain around your middle – and how, in the absence of scientific research into women's post-miscarriage bodies, we turned to forums and friends to see what is normal and what is not. As Jennie put it 'Things are often dismissed as "anecdotal", without a body of evidence to back it up, but lots of people reporting the same thing is not meaningless – whether it's been turned into a study or not.'

When I surveyed women, there was a lot of dissatisfaction about their postnatal bodies, but it was clear that this was in no small part down to how we, as a society, perceive women and mothers. Quite a few of the women yearned for not only greater acceptance of their new bodies, but also a wider recognition and respect for what their bodies had done. Whether it was growing one child, or five. Whether it was vaginal birth or caesarean. Whether they breastfed for three weeks or three years. Instead of becoming figures of fun for having drooping breasts, sagging stomachs and leaking when they coughed, these women needed to feel that the sacrifice they had made with their bodies was not only accepted, but appreciated. Many women found being bombarded by unrealistic post-baby bodies was detrimental to their self-worth and hindered their ability to accept their 'new me' – although many desperately wanted to do this. They craved an honest conversation about post-birth bodies, what to expect and what not to accept. They believe, as I do, that we deserve this.

Furthermore, the women I surveyed often knew *what* they needed to do to get back to optimal health (and I must stress again, that I do not mean 'getting thin' – I mean living in a body that feels comfortable and gives you the quality of life and longevity that you desire), but they did not feel supported to do so. Whether this had been trips to the GP where they had felt fobbed off and dismissed, or simply not being able to carve out time to visit a women's health physio or go to a gym, or for a swim; the over-riding themes that emerged were of women striving to heal, recover and create long-lasting changes but who were often falling at the first hurdle due to a lack of support. As I have said before, adding 'self-care' and 'get fit' to a woman's already over-flowing basket of *things to do*, without putting structures (or even just mind-shifts) in place to enable her to succeed, just creates an additional burden and more things to 'fail' at. As I have repeatedly said, we need a change in society. A society which recognises the physical feat of pregnancy, labour and early postpartum, respects it, and creates the environment in which women feel understood, nurtured and have the time and space to prioritise recovery.

While researching this book, I have heard such a wide array of symptoms/side-effects that women attribute to pregnancy and birth. Some make me laugh out loud, some make me wince, some make me pleased and hopeful, but many break my heart.

Some of what you will read below is distressing. Feel free to skip over bits you're not comfortable reading. Remember, this is not your story – they are theirs. Everybody is different. I have included a wide range of experiences in the hope that, if you are feeling alone and like you are the only one experiencing something, you will recognise yourself here. I also hope you will find inspiration in the case studies of women who have experienced some common postpartum issues – and overcome them.

## THE WEIRD

*'My feet have got bigger by half a size.'*

*'I was really gassy and my farts smelled like drains.'*

*'Sneeze farts are a thing! I hate sneezing but I have also developed hayfever and rhinitis – it came on and then stopped when my first baby was two, then it started again with my second baby'.*

*'I now have patches of darker hair on my legs.'*

*'My hair breaks more easily.'*

*'I used to hate cow's milk and wouldn't drink it in tea, but ever since I became pregnant with my first child I crave it – and now actually even drink a glass of it on its own, which would have made me retch pre-children... I am convinced it's something to do with calcium.'*

*'Loud, frequent (sometimes painful) hiccups which started in first pregnancy and haven't really stopped.'*

*'Farting from my vagina.'*

*'My hair has got darker.'*

*'Losing teeth!'*

*'The adhesions from my c-section pulled my bladder up into my uterus, and I would pee constantly or pee myself. They "cut it away" on my last baby and now my bladder is fine but the scar is like 20 inches deep into my stomach and then I have a belly popping over it.'*

*'My body did change shape – after two pregnancies very close together I became very thin (and not in a good way, I did not feel very healthy, in fact I felt depleted). Despite the weight loss, shirts that had fit me pre-pregnancy did not fit, as my rib cage*

*had definitely been pushed out.'*

*'Floaters in my eyes.'*

*'My joints ache quite a lot when getting up off the floor.'*

*'Larger breasts and enhanced sense of smell – both of which have stayed permanently!'*

*'Receding gums and I've had many trips to the dentist because of tooth pain.'*

*'More body hair!!'*

*'Strange mottling to the skin on my face that appeared during pregnancy and hasn't really gone away.'*

*'My poor vagina seems to have a tiny penis formed after the stitches.'*

*'My fingers swelled during pregnancy and haven't gone back to normal. I can't wear my engagement ring.'*

*'After my first child my left wrist became weak and "gave" at about 18 months postpartum for about a year. With my second child, it's 15 months postpartum and it's the right wrist.'*

## THE WONDERFUL

*'On the positive side I found I orgasm more quickly now, stupidly quickly soon after birth.'*

*'My breasts are bigger, but probably because of breastfeeding rather than pregnancy.'*

*'I discovered I'm pretty damned strong since having kids. I can rugby tackle a fully grown man, so I'd say that is new!'*

*'I used to get terrible migraines and cluster headaches almost weekly, and was on medication. I had to stop the medication*

*when I was pregnant with my first and I've never needed it again. Six years on and I can count on one hand the number of migraines I've had since.'*

*'Weirdly, having kids significantly improved my IBS. It was really quite life-changing for me – not as much need to plan trips around toilet proximity was liberating!'*

*'I had an inverted nipple pre-babies, and I was told I probably couldn't breastfeed but the greedy little sucker pulled my nipple out and fed successfully.'*

*'My periods are less painful.'*

*'I have better curves and bigger boobs! I was very thin before so quite happy about this!'*

*'I was lactose-intolerant before falling pregnant. Postpartum I wouldn't say I am completely cured, but I can have an ice cream now without any bad side effects.'*

*'Three pregnancies and two years of breastfeeding seems to have reversed my Polycystic Ovary Syndrome. I have fully-working cyst-free ovaries again.'*

*'My hair is thicker.'*

*'Before having my son I was short-sighted. Now I have perfect vision.'*

*'My periods changed, they got lighter.'*

## THE DISTRESSING

*'I had a back-to-back delivery and fractured my coccyx, which made it uncomfortable to sit for six weeks, making recovery and feeding incredibly difficult.'*

*'I had lots of migraines after both my children.'*

*'Sometimes during sex, I can feel where the scar is where I was stitched badly and it hurts.'*

*'My boobs no longer get excited during sex. This is hard for me as they were a big part of helping me orgasm.'*

*'The nerves in my stomach were damaged and I still have no feeling. I can't even properly feel if I am engaging my core.'*

*'Difficulty pooing as it seems to bypass the exit and needs to be helped out by digital manipulation through the vaginal wall. (I am so sorry)'*

*'I don't recognise my body anymore. My back is so weak and I am in pain all the time.'*

*'The post-birth stitches weren't done correctly so one of the labia on one side has a slit down which looks awful and I find it embarrassing.'*

*'Although luckily have not experienced faecal incontinence, I do feel a more urgent need to get to a toilet!'*

*'Developed fibroids which have led to heavier periods.'*

*'More intense cycles, not just periods but severe ovulation pain which I didn't notice much before and more intense PMT (very irritable, teary, painful cramps, back pain and headaches).'*

*'The way I look "downstairs" has changed for the worse and it has definitely had a negative impact on my sex life and sexual confidence.'*

*'I'm very run down. I keep getting recurrent mastitis which makes me pretty much unable to function until the antibiotics kick in.'*

*'The c-section scar tissue damage hurts and is sore. I have been for a scan and need to decide whether to have surgery.'*

## 'WHAT DO YOU WISH YOU HAD KNOWN IN ADVANCE OR SOMEONE HAD TOLD YOU?'

*'I didn't know that I'd be slightly more incontinent with urine, despite having a c-section. I didn't know that this would still be affected.'*

*'The weight of pregnancy and its long-term impact on the pelvic girdle.'*

*'I wish there was less of a taboo about discussing these issues. Like, I had no idea I would bleed heavily for six weeks after and then immediately start my periods again – in spite of exclusively breastfeeding.'*

*'I wish someone had told me about the hair loss. It came out in handfuls and was pretty alarming at first.'*

*'I wish I'd known more about how hard it could be to establish breastfeeding. When I started feeding my eldest the pain was excruciating – I had flat nipples and needed shields for the first few weeks to feed without pain. And then stopping feeding was hard too, and massively hit my mood with all the hormonal changes.'*

*'I wish I had truly understood impact of an emergency c-section and the consequences of not prioritising recovery, even when you have a toddler! Also, I was deeply embarrassed by the urinary incontinence and wish I'd known how common that is!'*

*'I remember being shocked at the blood loss after the birth – no one talks about it prior. I bought one pack of maternity pads to take to the hospital with me – ha! I was going through one pack every two days for three months!'*

*'I wish I'd been told "you don't have to live with this" – stop trying to sell me incontinence pads and start talking about therapies!'*

'I wish I had never used sugar to fuel me and slept instead of trying to half-arsedly clean a kitchen while exhausted.'

'I wish I'd known that most of the things that bother me now (varicose veins and stretch marks, and lack of sleep) you can't actually control or prevent. A lot is either hereditary or down to luck and the kind of child you have. I'm naturally a control freak, so it was hard for me to feel like I'd failed.'

'I wish there was more acceptance and honesty. Some social awareness of the stress and trauma it puts on your body. Stop celebrating "just getting on with it".'

'I wish I'd had information, before giving birth, about what to expect after. We talk lots about what goes in your hospital bag but how embarrassing to ask your husband to buy haemorrhoid cream because you need some today, not delivered in 3–5 days!'

'I had a big fat baby in my short body and my stomach muscles were shot to bits. No advice on how to help it or correct it despite it being noticed at a six-week check.'

'Better clarity on timescales and how long recovery takes. I would query that you can "get your body back". I think a big missing piece of the narrative is supporting women to understand that their bodies are forever changed.'

'How hypermobility would affect pregnancy, childbirth and my pelvic organ issues.'

'I know friends in France and Germany who have given birth have automatically been referred to a women's physio to check pelvic floor function and strength. That would have been really useful.'

'Motherhood makes you use your body in a totally different way to how you used to, and it literally happens overnight. I would pay to learn how to get my body back to health.'

When you search forums and feeds (sometimes called 'doom scrolling') you can come across some very bleak outcomes for postnatal women and it can make you feel hopeless. However, with a more open environment to talk about these things, and with a growing interest and expertise (only about a millennium overdue!) in women's health, things are improving, and I am now more frequently hearing better recovery stories. Also note that the scores of women who have experienced gentle births and full, or simple, recoveries will likely not have answered my call for quotes and stories. As I will expand on in the next chapter, although weird, wonderful and distressing things *do* happen, most will likely not happen to you.

I spoke to 10 women in depth about their journeys back to health after postpartum physical issues. All these women have overcome significant challenges and I hope you find some inspiration and motivation from their stories.

## CASE STUDIES
### Natalie Dale

I first encountered Natalie when she contacted us about providing information for the case we were taking to Parliament about how underfunding in postnatal care was having an adverse impact on the health of new mothers. Natalie had had a pretty traumatic forceps birth, which ended up with her baby in NICU and her dealing with a third-degree tear. When Natalie got in touch, she was reeling from a diagnosis of prolapse and struggling with PTSD from her birth experience. What was very clear from her message was that she was passionate about helping other women and trying to ensure no other woman had to go through what she went through. Natalie has spent the last few years not only healing herself, but sharing her healing journey online and specialising as a pre- and postnatal yoga and Pilates instructor, so that she can help others. Suffice to say, she is an inspiration. She now has two sons (Ethan and Sebastian) and is in rude health. But a few years ago, she had become so low after the trauma of her birth had been dismissed by the hospital, and alongside coming to terms with the prolapse diagnosis, that she felt suicidal. I am glad that Natalie felt able to share this very personal part of her story as I know that many other women go through similar feelings

– indeed, the Bits of Me podcast recently demonstrated that 30–40% of women with severe tears feel like their baby 'would be better off without them'. When I was researching women's stories for our Parliamentary campaign, this sentiment – the feeling of not being able to go on – came up often and was often directly related to adverse physical outcomes after birth.

Natalie told me how she saw several healthcare professionals, including a private obstetrician-gynaecologist, who made her feel worse about her prolapse. They gave her no hope of healing or recovery. She was told that it would never improve and that she would not be able to run, practice her beloved yoga or even poo normally ever again. As a 35-year-old woman who was used to running marathons, she found this devastating. Natalie was not only determined that this was not going to be the end of the things she loved, but she also felt she knew and trusted her body more than the healthcare professionals who she felt were writing her off. She was lucky to have the time and resources to be able to create her own care pathway, by seeking private help both from a women's health physio and a counsellor. We both despaired, as she recounted her story, that the waiting list for a woman openly talking about suicidal thoughts was 12 months! However, in tandem, these women that she found (she went through a few therapists at first, as is often the case, to find the right 'fit') helped Natalie piece herself back together. After initially being told she had a Grade 2 prolapse, Natalie was given a better diagnosis from her physio, stating it was a Grade 1, but it did include all of her pelvic organs. Natalie admitted to me that she had become 'obsessed' with monitoring her prolapse by looking at it and feeling it when she wiped. This 'obsession' paid dividends by the time she had healed though, as it was clear to her that it had, indeed, disappeared as her physio told her it had. There is scant research on complete healing of a prolapse, but at least two trials[78] show that significant 'reversal' or reduction in symptoms is possible with pelvic floor muscle training and lifestyle modifications.

After hitting rock bottom and suffering with intense physical and emotional side-effects from prolapse, Natalie was able – through dedicated training – to completely eliminate her symptoms and now lives symptom-free. She went on to have another child (via planned caesarean section) and she can run, do yoga, have a normal sex life, lift heavy things – she can even lift both of her sons and run – with no impact. I am hoping that if you have just received a diagnosis of prolapse, that this will be the positive news you need to hear. Natalie sometimes experiences pelvic tightness – especially if she has been doing lots of squats. For this she uses a 'wand' to massage the internal scar tissue from her third-degree tear. She also uses a technique called 'hypopressives' (exercises which retrain the core and reduce internal pressure) but has stressed to me that you really need to first work with a practitioner to ensure you have the technique right as it is not easy, and the wrong technique could make symptoms worse.

I asked Natalie for any tips she would give to mothers in a similar position to her. She says: firstly, if you are unfortunate enough to end up in NICU and you have a bad tear, you could make frozen maxi pads with added aloe vera to help numb the area as you move from the car to the ward. You could also take cold packs or heat packs if you have had a caesarean. Natalie echoes Sam Harrison's advice to take cushions to make yourself more comfortable, ask for a reclining chair if there is one and ask for as much help as you need. It is not being a nuisance to ask for help.

Secondly, Natalie says, reach out for help and keep reaching even if the first people you encounter are not ready or able to help you. Physical ailments can, obviously, have emotional and psychological ramifications. When Natalie was really struggling, and on a really long waiting list for mental health support, she reached out to PANDAS (Postnatal Depression Awareness and Support) and found their helpline to be 'incredible.' The helpline is open 11am–10pm every day and it is free (see the Resources at the back of the book). Natalie found peer support from others who had been through similar experiences particularly helpful. She was keen to stress how helpful it is to share the experience of prolapse with someone else. She happened to have someone in her NCT group who was also suffering and willing to talk openly (not too unusual considering the statistics!) Why Mums Don't Jump podcast creator, Helen Ledwick, also facilitates mums with prolapse connecting and helping each other.

Natalie advises staying off Google (if you can!) as it can really send you on a downward spiral. Rather, look at well-respected experts in the field and the free resources they provide to help women in your situation. She cites Femme Fusion Fitness and women's health physio Jennifer Constable on Instagram as two such examples.

Lastly, Natalie emphasises that you often need to be a strong advocate for yourself. If the first healthcare professional you see dismisses you, or you don't get the results you want, then keep going. Ask for second opinions, ask for referrals you think you need, try to be assertive. Nobody knows your body like you do and you deserve to recover.

### Lucy Hawes

'This is fucking crazy, you really shouldn't' is not the way that you imagine a first session with any kind of health practitioner would go, but that's the reaction Lucy Hawes (a project director in Dubai) got when she announced to her new women's health physio that she would be running the London marathon just five months after the birth of her second son. However, Jade Lucas-Read quickly had the measure of Lucy and said, 'but, I kind of get the impression you're going to do it anyway, so we've got work to do!' Lucy says that she knew from that first expletive that this was a woman she could work with.

I feel like this case study should come with a warning: don't try this at home, kids. But, actually, I am kind of fed up of women being told 'don't do this anymore' after having children, especially if it's the thing that makes you feel like who you are and gets you through the day. Yes, you perhaps need to have a better understanding of your body, and how to not totally fuck it up, but there needs to be a balance. One where you can still do the things you used to do and feel like you again, as well as maintaining physical integrity. Lucy needed something that would make her feel more than 'just' (it's never 'just', by the way!) a mother. She needed something of her old life. At this point, I should point out that Lucy is very much a Type A personality. I have known Lucy since our university days (she got a First, obviously) and she is a very driven, committed and goal-orientated person. She also recognises that she has the means to be able to work with someone privately and intensively, which is just not possible for many of us. She was able to form a real partnership with Jade in order to meet her goal: to run the London marathon 'dry' and without pain and discomfort.

Lucy had run her first marathon a year after giving birth to her first son and she describes it as 'horrible'. She was not able to run for a great deal of it as she had intense pain in her hip and her iliotibial (IT) band down the side of her leg. She puts this down to a compromised pelvic floor. She also had to wear continence pads and says she was 'wet the whole way'. Leaking urine on runs had really got to Lucy. She felt embarrassed and depressed. She had not heard about women's health physios after her first son and so had gone straight from running 5km to marathons without that kind of support. She also continued running through her next pregnancy. She feels that this all contributed, along with internal scarring, to her continence issues. Under the supervision of her 'partner-in-quim', Jade, she started gentle Pilates and had both manual and electrode manipulation/stimulation of her vagina, as well as manual techniques to help with her slight diastasis recti. Eventually, after about eight weeks, she was 'allowed' to do gentle runs, but Jade suggested she use a pessary called a 'contiform' to help support her pelvic organs. Lucy had a degree of prolapse that needed support while she ran. She told me that, although helpful for adding extra support, the actual logistics of fitting in runs, with kids and work, is hard enough without 'Shoving something up your fanny! It's not easy to do. It's tricky! And you've got the kids banging on the bathroom door. You're knackered. Sometimes I'd be in tears. But you keep going.'

When Lucy ran her second marathon, it was a completely different experience to the first. I could see when I spoke to her how healing it had been for her to achieve such a feat – to feel physically fit and at her peak even after children. She ran the whole way in her second marathon and her time was an hour faster than her first attempt. In addition, while she was reluctant to go to a gym or train in a group before she partnered with Jade, for fear of wetting herself and feeling humiliated, she can now happily take part in group activities. She also no longer needs to rely on a pessary, as she has managed to strengthen her pelvic muscles to such a degree that her prolapse is asymptomatic, if not wholly reversed.

Lucy is aware of her limits, though. She knows there are certain exercises she can't do (intense jumping) and so she avoids them. She also knows that if her scar tissue gets too tight then she might experience leaking again when coughing or sneezing. If this happens she either makes an appointment to see Jade for manual release or she does it herself with her 'wand'. Lucy is keen to point out that women should not assume it is pelvic floor *weakness* that is making them leak. Too-tight pelvic floor muscles and scar tissue can also have a negative impact. Lucy said to me, 'It's a maintenance thing now. It's for life but I'm not prepared to accept leaking as part and parcel of being a mum.'

I was so impressed with Lucy's story. The tenacity it would take to tackle a marathon, at any time, let alone in the early postpartum days, is awesome. It's not for me, but it does make me think – well what *is* there that I really want to do that I'm not up to fitness-wise at the moment? I used to love big hiking trips overseas and Lucy's story makes me think – maybe I *could* get back to that... and maybe I *should*. Would I worry about there not being enough accessible toilets if I took off on an intrepid adventure? If that's the case, then I need to get myself to a state of pelvic fitness and confidence in order to remove that barrier. It's confidence that has been Lucy's biggest prize. The confidence to go out for a run, or to a class and not to have to worry about leaking or damaging her pelvic health.

Lucy's candour is also admirable. She told me that a friend's husband had done a double-take on hearing her speak about leaking, but, as Lucy says 'This is the reality. We shouldn't feel ashamed.' Lucy said she feels that being open, both about your issues and what you want to achieve, will help you overcome any obstacles. She is passionate that women insist that their GP refer them to women's health physios so that they can really get to know their bodies. And, lastly, she reflects that we ought to work on all the bits of our body – as a strong body will help you compensate for areas that may have been compromised in pregnancy and childbirth. Hear, hear.

### Grace Pearson

Grace Pearson is a youth minister's wife and lives in Cambridgeshire with her husband and two young sons. She struggled significantly after the birth of her first son, as an undetected UTI led to sepsis and, in parallel, very severe mastitis. When we speak, she tells me that, although full recovery took time, it was her faith, good support, and an outlook that framed this period as 'just a moment in time' rather than something that had been irrevocably damaging, that helped her recover and thrive.

Grace had a second-degree tear with Andrew, her firstborn, and was really struggling to pass urine while still in the hospital. The pain was so bad that she would have to shower to be able to go at all. Despite raising the issue a few times, midwives told her it was just stinging from the tear and would settle down. It didn't though. On day 4, at home, her community midwife told her to 'put some Vaseline on her bits' and told her that she was 'fine'. She wasn't. Later that day, her husband realised that something was going very wrong. For someone who was 'usually horizontally laid-back' Grace was becoming agitated at having guests in her home and when Ben went to find her upstairs, she was shivering and unable to move or speak properly. They went to the doctors who also quickly realised that Grace was not doing well at all, and an ambulance was called. Grace's heartrate was very high and she could not hold Andrew to feed him. She arrived at hospital four hours later. Unfortunately, diagnosis, treatment and care were all poor from this point on, partly because she was falling between several different therapeutic areas. Grace's leaking breasts were bound with gauze in A&E, instead of her being helped to feed or express. This led to blocked ducts which caused double mastitis. Grace was in intensive care for eight days, during which baby Andrew was mostly bottle fed. She laments how this affected her breastfeeding journey and bonding, as Andrew could have been held to her breast. As it was, she was trying to express in the first few days but could barely hold the pump and found only pus coming out. When she came out of hospital she suffered night terrors and developed an abscess in one breast. Luckily, she was able to have access to a wonderful NHS lactation consultant (funding for whom has since been cut) who helped her on a daily basis with relactation (resuming breastfeeding after a period of not being able to do so) and clearing the abscess. Grace cannot speak highly enough of the help she received via this free specialist breastfeeding support service, and also the help of close friends.

Grace went on to breastfeed (though not exclusively) for another five months, although she was plagued with recurrent mastitis. She imagines the scarring that occurred from the first, very severe, bout played a part in this – but she also discovered that she was wearing the wrong size nipple shields (sometimes called a 'flange'… truly) when expressing. She found that she was using a size too big which was causing trauma to her breast tissue, and when she swapped for the correct size she no longer had issues with mastitis. However, she didn't feel like she had recovered fully from all of the physical trauma until she stopped breastfeeding at five months. This was a bittersweet moment. While she began to regain a sense of her 'old self' by going out running and the night terrors stopping, alongside being free of mastitis and the recurrent UTIs she'd been having, she also felt like she'd failed. In addition to societal and family pressure, she found it mentally challenging not to be providing breastmilk for her baby. But her husband told her that 'her colour' had come back and she felt like she finally had the chance to heal.

When Grace fell pregnant again, she was concerned about history repeating itself as she began suffering with UTIs again. Her biggest fear was having to go into hospital to be treated but, because the UK was in 'lockdown' because of Covid-19, she was treated at home with the strongest antibiotics that could be prescribed. She describes her second birth, with son Greig, as 'positive'. She birthed in an upright position as she knows she has an inverted coccyx from a mountain biking accident and felt this would help make things easier. As it was, she had no tearing – despite the baby being over 9lb. And, although she did get a urine infection again in the postpartum period, she was able to get rid of it without having to be readmitted to hospital. Grace was also able to exclusively breastfeed Greig, which was something she was unsure would be possible after her earlier experience. She has not had a recurrence of mastitis, and she thinks this is down to all the support she received with positioning while feeding Andrew and using the correct 'flange' (is it just me, or is that the weirdest name ever for an object? It has overtones of Phoebe Buffet*) when expressing.

When I asked Grace about how other mothers could try to cope in similar circumstances, she said 'Be prepared to battle. You know your

---

* *Friends* sitcom reference

body. No one should feel like an idiot for saying something is wrong.' She was also keen that we are not 'too British about things' and are prepared to be vulnerable. She says she was much happier to 'stand up for herself' the second time around and had no trouble going into the maternity centre if she felt concerned about anything. Grace says she is still learning to set boundaries, but saying 'no family' in the early days so that she could establish breastfeeding in a relaxed, intimate environment was a real help. Having said that, she has been lucky to have a lot of support from friends, family and the community and was surprised and grateful to have had 'no baby blues' the second time around.

Grace had this advice for women going through bouts of mastitis: 'I experienced four episodes of mastitis with my first child who I combination fed for five months. I have now been exclusively breastfeeding my second for eight months and not had a single episode or lack of milk production. Mastitis doesn't mean you can't do it, but it is the biggest challenge I think you will ever face when breastfeeding. Support is key. Medical – make sure you get antibiotics ASAP. Physical – ring your health visitor. Find a feeding specialist to come and check your latch. Emotional – ask for help. You don't need to be dealing with everything else. Focus on skin-to-skin and rest. Find someone to talk to. It does get better (please believe me even when you can't see through the pain) and it doesn't need to dictate your feeding journey but support is key. Don't suffer in silence'.

### Kim Vopni

Kim is one of the experts I turned to when I began writing this book. She had been a shining beacon of no-nonsense-nunny-info for me since I had my first son. She goes by the name of The Vagina Coach and she confided in me how difficult it was to take the decision to have surgery for her prolapsed rectum (rectocele), in light of the years she had spent investing in not only her own pelvic health, but that of scores of other women through her work as a personal trainer and pelvic health specialist. But not all pelvic health issues can be addressed in the same way. Pelvic floor physio, Pilates and hypopressives, among other treatments and training, can work absolute wonders for some people, but it is not a one-size-fits-all solution. Kim had spent almost a decade trying to alleviate the symptoms of her prolapse and had, indeed, already been successful in reversing her uterine prolapse – but a rectocele can be a trickier beast. Kim found that pelvic health physios she spoke with agreed with her that a rectocele can be more difficult to manage with conservative measures.

On top of that, Kim had been battling for a number of years with an autoimmune condition called Hashimoto's. Hashimoto's damages the thyroid gland and can cause fatigue, constipation, heavy and irregular periods and anxiety/depression – among other symptoms. It can also be a frustratingly long wait for a diagnosis, as it was for Kim. Kim feels that the constipation that accompanied her autoimmune condition was a big factor in her developing a rectocele despite her obvious dedication to health, fitness and the integrity and strength of her pelvic floor. She also found, more than a decade after her first birth, that she had almost certainly had a partial levator ani avulsion (which is when part of your pelvic floor muscles tear away from the bone) which could also have contributed to the rectocele, and/or uterine prolapse as they are indicated in prolapse prevalence. Kim is reassuringly positive about both her birth experiences, but she feels her first birth (in which her baby came out sideways) may have caused the levator ani damage and she also suffered with extremely painful haemorrhoids afterwards, which made her feel fearful of her second birth. She had been contemplating a planned caesarean but, in the end, opted for an epidural which eased the pushing stage and meant she did not have a repeat of the excruciating piles the second time around.

Kim has successfully sent her Hashimoto's into remission, by focusing on her stress levels, gut health and digestion. When her Hashimoto's came under control, she stopped suffering with constipation and heavy periods and became asymptomatic with her rectocele. However, she began to notice symptoms again around two years ago, which she equates with ageing, declining oestrogen levels and her stress levels rising as the Covid-19 pandemic began to loom. It was at this point that she decided her mental health could not take dealing with the day-to-day discomfort and anxiety that her rectocele caused. Kim's decision to undergo surgery came after she had reached the end of her tether dealing with the daily discomfort and burden of living with a rectocele. She told me that she felt constantly as if she had poo in her rectum ('I was literally full of shit!') later in the day if she had not had successful bowel movements. She was upset that she could not have spontaneous sex, or even commit to exercise and evening activities with friends, and this negatively impacted her mental and physical health. She said that if she had to lean over to pick something up, she would do an awkward side-bend with her knees together as she was afraid that 'something would come out' if she squatted or leaned over. I had never heard someone speak so openly about what it felt like to have a prolapse. Obviously, this is particular to a rectocele, and to Kim herself, but she told me that she felt a constant need to poo but without the urge and she also felt a constant bulge in her vagina like there was 'something in there'. She also felt vulnerable and that she didn't want to 'have *anything* going in me'. This all sounds like it would dramatically impact your freedom, confidence and quality of life, not to mention your mental health.

Kim's openness about her symptoms, and also about going for surgery, has been so refreshing. While women are beginning to talk more freely about prolapse, surgery still seems like a 'taboo' area that we don't talk about. This blank space, about what happens when pelvic floor rehabilitation doesn't work, needs filling. Which is where Kim steps in. And brilliantly so. Kim is keen to point out that on this journey, the 'fix' doesn't begin and end with surgery. She tried the more conservative treatments (and, I mean, if anyone is going to have road-tested these options to the hilt, it's The Vagina Coach) and in the end, it wasn't enough to cure her prolapse and give her the quality of life she needed and deserved. And so, Kim researched her options, decided on native-tissue surgery, and to have the surgery now before the menopause hit and potentially weakened the tissue in her vagina. She supplemented with bio-identical hormones and used local vaginal oestrogen to enable her to feel like her vaginal tissue was prepped for surgery. The surgery was in November 2020 and Kim is making an excellent recovery. She is very clear with me that surgery doesn't 'fix' you – it gives you a starting place to build on and maintain, to be used *in addition* to optimising your digestion and strengthening your pelvic floor. She created her own care pathway of both 'prehab' and 'rehab', which she chronicles in depth on her Instagram and blog. My favourite two take-aways from her blog were: she took a husband-sized dildo to her surgery with her so that the surgeon did not 'over-correct', which would lead to painful sex (having winced at accounts of the so-called 'husband stitch' regarding post-birth repairs, I think this is genius!); and treating her rehab like she would a postpartum period – with rest, healing self-care and gradual strengthening exercises.

It was lovely to hear Kim talk about how much more confidence and freedom of movement she has experienced after surgery, as well as being able to have more freedom with fitness as well as sex with her husband (whom she credits as being very supportive). What is striking is how she overcame a sense of shame that she experienced both in opting for surgery and then talking about it, particularly as someone within the pelvic health community. 'The truth is, sometimes surgery is the best option'. This echoes something women's health physio Elaine Miller told me. That, for some, pelvic floor physio is enough and for others surgery will be necessary – if not immediately, then further down the line. I agree wholeheartedly with Kim that we need to remove the shame around that. Kim will also be helping a broader community of women now by recounting her rehabilitation journey, to show how putting your body in the best shape possible, and taking the time to recover properly, will increase chances of a successful surgery and pay dividends for your long-term health.

### Kat Thomas

Kat is a Fanny Crusader. After having a 'horrendous' first birth experience, in which she had a borderline third- to fourth-degree tear, followed by a healing planned caesarean birth, Kat is now starting her career as a midwife, with a passion for perineal health. When I spoke to Kat, having met her through my son's nursery, she filled me with hope about the future of midwifery as her passion for women's health and bodily autonomy and integrity was palpable. 'I want women to feel safe and cared for', she told me. 'I don't want women to feel unimportant and that what happens to their bodies doesn't matter.' Kat is determined to be part of a change in midwifery, which – although it often offers outstanding care, can sometimes leave postpartum women feeling like an afterthought. Kat experienced first-hand the type of poor care that she doesn't want to be responsible for giving; she felt abandoned throughout her first labour and a subsequent six-hour wait to be taken to theatre and sutured after a severe tear. Kat wants to make sure that women in her care will never feel how she felt.

The impact of the poor care she received, and the third-degree tear (just a 'paper thin wall' before it was a fourth-degree tear), was significant for Kat's physical and mental health. She suffered with postnatal depression and felt she struggled to bond with her baby as 'that association with pain' was there. This was exacerbated by breastfeeding '24/7' in a sitting-down position, while in intense pain, as well as poor follow-up from the hospital and community midwives. When Kat complained of a stubborn stitch that she could feel high up near her cervix, she was brushed off. Eventually it dissolved but she felt similarly neglected after a referral for women's physio that had been promised at her six-week check up with an obstetrician/gynaecologist (this check-up is standard after a third or fourth-degree tear) failed to materialise. She did not feel strong enough at the time to pursue the referral and so it was six months before she began to 'rehabilitate' her pelvic floor. She did this by researching online how to train her pelvic floor muscles and using the Squeezy app. She was pretty gung-ho at first, doing this daily but, eventually, the enthusiasm dwindled and she did it more ad hoc. Her early commitment paid off, as she does not now experience any continence issues – although she admitted to me that she wouldn't like to be tested on a trampoline. I mean, who would?

Kat's main issue with recovery was how it affected her sex life. There was both a mental and physical block to her and her husband getting back to having enjoyable sex. She didn't try sex until six months postpartum and found it painful for at least a year from that point. She became so worried that it was taking so long to feel normal that this created more tension in her body, which added to the pain. It was a vicious circle. Kat feels like this lack of intimacy definitely affected their relationship, despite her husband being very understanding. Kat told me that giving herself time and taking it slow was the key to resolving this issue for them. She said they 'started again at the beginning' and when I probed further (like you do with a new mum friend you met at the nursery gates – ha!), asking if she meant they started with petting like teenagers – she said yes, and that they built on that and used lots of lubrication. This tallies with what Sam Evans said: taking it slow, doing what you're comfortable with and not putting the whole emphasis on penetrative sex. This paced approach worked for Kat and her husband and they have got back to where they both want to be with their sex life.

Kat and I talked about scar manipulation and how that could perhaps further enhance her long-term recovery and health. She was really interested in it and shocked that this type of information wasn't readily available during her midwifery training. I told Kat about how my early scar manipulation has (I think!) helped me regain all of the sensation in the skin around my c-section scar and she was amazed as she still experiences numbness around her scar. We also talked about how scar tissue can impact you internally and she asked me for some research papers. I have no doubt that this will now also influence Kat's approach to women postnatally. She already impresses upon them how early pelvic floor exercises can help blood flow and healing for the vaginal/perineal tissue and I am sure she will do her research and learn about the impact of scar release. I left the interview (okay, it might have been coffee and a right natter at our local café – bliss) by telling Kat that midwifery is lucky to have her. So many women will benefit from her approach of putting women first. A fanny crusader indeed.

### Anya Hayes

I met Anya Hayes, an awesome multi-hyphenate if ever there was one (combining motherhood with an editorial job, writing books about women's health and being a Pilates instructor) at a book launch for Rebecca Schiller's awesome pregnancy guide *Your No Guilt Pregnancy Plan*. I was aware that Anya had suffered some complications as a result of her births and was keen to find out more about her situation and recovery.

Anya has two boys, Maurice and Freddie; both abdominal births. Her first caesarean had been what is called a 'crash' emergency c-section, which is when there is deemed to be immediate threat to the life of the mother or baby. After a long and difficult labour, Anya was rushed to theatre as Maurice was not doing well. Anya's recovery was difficult; as well as the pain from the c-section scar, she became very depleted which meant that she ended up suffering with anaemia and a really bad chest infection.

New motherhood can render even the most well intentioned and knowledgeable woman incapable of putting herself first when she needs to. Anya not only battled through significant scar pain (and pain related to adhesions), but also 'just kept going' through a traumatic miscarriage experience which led to her being hospitalised abroad with issues from 'retained tissue'. This was an experience which, she says, made her even more grateful for our NHS. Anya had been to see a GP about her continuing c-section scar pain at about nine months postpartum but, without palpating (physically touching) the scar, he declared that all was fine as she did not have an infection. It was not until the birth of her second son, Freddie, who came along after she had experienced one further pregnancy loss, that she realised the extent of what was happening with her scar. The right side of her scar had been particularly sore and her clinical notes explained that this was because there had been a vertical incision here as well as a horizontal incision. This 'T-shape' incision is not uncommon for emergency caesareans as it creates a larger opening from which to get the baby out quickly and safely. The vertical incision scar was not visible on the surface, as it was a deeper, uterine incision, but this explained the nagging pain that Anya had experienced since Maurice's birth.

Anya had a planned caesarean with her second son, which, although a much calmer experience, took a great deal longer than she had envisaged. Once Freddie had been born, the surgeon was able to tell Anya that the reason the procedure had taken so long was because 'she had never seen so much scar tissue'. Indeed, the surgeon was able to cut away some of the excess tissue and rectify some of the adhesions before sewing Anya's stomach back up. Anya found this scar, although tender initially, much easier to heal from. Aesthetically, Anya describes this scar as 'gliding along the first; a calm, almost invisible white line, while its predecessor zigzags up and up and down angrily around it. [The second scar is] a testament to its much more serene and peaceful story.' Although you can have surgery to remove excessive scar tissue/deal with adhesions, Anya advises that you proceed with caution as you could actually end up creating more scar tissue, which would just make things worse. While it is worth exploring, a more conservative approach is probably the best course initially.

Anya found out about scar manipulation after seeking help from her friend, a women's health physio called Emma Brockwell, for shoulder pain. Emma had advised Anya that improving the strength in her glutes and massaging her scar would help alleviate the shoulder pain – which it did. Anya told me that she feels very lucky to have had a friend point her in the right direction, as scar tissue can 'impact so much of your general strength and function'. Two years after Freddie was born, Anya went to another pelvic health physio, Clare Bourne, for treatment. Even though this was eight years after her first abdominal birth, the difference this made to Anya's comfort levels and mobility cannot be underestimated. As a Pilates teacher she was really aware of movements she could no longer do and a constant hip pain that she feels is absolutely the result of adhesions. As well as visiting Clare for scar manipulation, she also practices it regularly on herself at least every other day.

For mothers who are experiencing 'unexplained' pain and mobility issues after a caesarean, Anya implores you 'not to be fobbed off' and also not to give up on yourself. She feels you sometimes have to be tenacious to get the care and treatment you deserve. She also advises you to get curious about your body and look into things yourself, stating 'Sometimes, you have to somewhat lead the charge. I know that that is particularly hard if it comes at a time when you feel exhausted and vulnerable, like a lot of new mothers, but it can help avoid a health crisis which could make you feel even worse. You have to live in your body forever.'

Anya credits journaling (where you write your thoughts down, often daily) and writing blogs as being a helpful outlet in her recovery. She also found connecting with others, through the Make Birth Better organisation, hugely helpful. Beyond that, she says that swimming, practising yoga and 'self-compassion mindfulness' helped on her recovery journey. Anya also completed a triathlon six months after Freddie was born which she says 'was a bit silly in hindsight, but sort of restored my "faith" and pride in my body a bit'.

## Sabrina Sweeney

Sabrina lives in my home town. We met while out on a climate change rally, both in the early days of pregnancy. I was further along and had told Sabrina I was pregnant but she was a few weeks behind me and, although she wanted to let on, she held her news back. We next saw each other when our tummies had swollen and we excitedly planned postpartum coffee-shop trips and the like, blissfully unaware of what the next year had in store for us. It was 2020, and although there were rumblings about a new virus in China, we were not in any way prepared for how different the world would look in just a few short weeks. I had a cuppa with Sabrina in a local café a couple of weeks before my second son was born and then I didn't see her again until our babies were three months old – and even then, we had to be outside and at the requisite two-metre distance from each other (due to 'social distancing' measures). It was a far cry from my first postpartum experience of meeting up with NCT mums on the regular and discussing every ache, pain, and concern.

So, I didn't actually find out until I was writing this book that Sabrina had had a postdural puncture (see p20) after having her daughter. I was running my interview questions past Sabrina, as she is a journalist and I was nervous about interviewing some of the other journalists for this book, when she said 'well, I had a postdural puncture, if you want to hear about that.' As it was something I had written about for the book, but hadn't heard of anyone having, I thought it would be an important aspect to cover.

Sabrina had her first daughter, Aéla, by caesarean section five years earlier. It had been a planned section as she suffered an internal carotid artery dissection (a tear in the inner layer of the wall of a carotid artery), a few months before becoming pregnant. She was advised against a vaginal delivery by her medical team as pushing during labour (the Valsalva manoeuvre) would put too much pressure on her arteries and could lead to complications including stroke. One of the symptoms of the dissection is an extreme headache, so when Sabrina started experiencing a bad headache after the birth of her second child, Saibh, she was concerned she had dissected again.

However, as she gave birth three days into the 2020 UK lockdown, things were pretty chaotic at the London hospital. She did not receive an answer from the nurse who had gone off to enquire whether a consultant could see her, and in fact she never saw that nurse again. No visitors were allowed (birth partners were, frustratingly, considered visitors) overnight. She found that she was either left alone for long periods of time or that several midwives would check on her in quick succession. It was disorientating, lonely and difficult. Sabrina had to leave her baby alone as she went to the toilet 'peeing blood' and her over-riding memory is of packing her bag herself, very carefully and cautiously so as not to tear her stitches, to leave. She felt she just had to get out of the hospital. The car journey back to Whitstable was long and painful. 'You cannot describe how painful that car journey is after a c-section, you feel every bump'. Throughout the journey, her headache worsened and when she got home she was barely able to move, so her husband and father 'sort of dragged' her into the house.

By the next morning her headache had got so bad that she could not sit up. Sabrina suffered with migraines anyway, but told me this pain was different and felt 'like my head was exploding'. If she needed to use the toilet, she would have to keep her head tilted backwards as she could not be upright. She also experienced balance and hearing issues, such as feeling like the room was swirling, and hearing echoes and reverberations. She didn't know what was wrong with her, but didn't believe it was her dissection condition because she didn't have the accompanying symptoms of a droopy eyelid and shrinking pupil. Eventually, a Google search in the early hours suggested that it could be a 'postdural puncture'. When Sabrina relayed her birth experience to me, it was clear that the epidural procedure had been quite literally hit and miss, as it had taken 20 minutes, and two anaesthetists, to administer. Finally, with something of an explanation, Sabrina was able to get her husband to call the hospital and she was immediately transferred over to the anaesthetist who kept in regular contact over the coming days. Sabrina was extremely anxious about having to go back into hospital (never great in any circumstances postpartum, but at the height of a pandemic that was causing serious issues in our hospitals, this was more than understandable) but, luckily, the anaesthetist had a simple suggestion, which worked. Caffeine. This 'increases cerebral vasoconstriction by blocking adenosine receptors and leads to augmented CSF production by stimulating sodium-potassium pumps',[79] which means it can reduce blood flow, leading to an increase of your cerebral spinal fluid (CSF) which provides a cushioning effect around your brain, therefore lessening pain. This helps to resolve the headache, but you may also need a 'blood patch' if you still experience symptoms. Sabrina was really grateful that there was something she could try at home to alleviate her extreme discomfort. Mindful that she was breastfeeding an infant and didn't want her baby ingesting too much caffeine, she started sipping on green tea and, luckily, found relief. In fact, from that moment on – with maintaining rest and regularly drinking other fluids as well as caffeine – her headache began to dissipate. By the sixth day postpartum, it was gone.

Sabrina has had no long-term ill effects from the postdural puncture, but she wishes she had been better prepared for it. In ordinary times, being able to have her birth partner with her in hospital, she might have stayed in for longer and the problem could have been rectified in hospital. She's adamant that this simple solution to something so debilitating should be common knowledge. Sabrina feels lucky, because she had no problems bonding or breastfeeding, despite the awful headache, but she cites the support of her family for this. She was able to breastfeed lying prone and her family looked after her eldest child so that she could rest. If this happened to someone without a similar support structure, it could really negatively affect their postpartum experience. If Sabrina were to offer any advice to a woman experiencing this, then it would be to demand to see a consultant if you are feeling very poorly postpartum. She wishes she had been a better advocate for herself. Obviously, it's much easier to see this in hindsight, as when you are in the midst of something as personally seismic as having a baby, at the same time as something as globally colossal as a deadly pandemic, and you are left alone with no support system, I think you can be forgiven for mustering your last bit of energy to pack your bags and go home.

It is worth noting that if caffeine does not provide immediate relief then you need to flag this with your healthcare provider, as severe headaches postpartum can require urgent attention.

## Helen Russell

Helen Russell is used to being candid about her life, as a journalist and as someone who deep dives into what makes us tick as humans for her (bestselling) books. I knew before I spoke to her that her road to becoming a mother had been bumpy, with many years, and pounds, spent on IVF – alongside other complementary fertility treatments. When we spoke, she was equally open about her birth experiences: 'Terrible! There's no easy way to get a baby out.' So it is not surprising that she describes motherhood as not only her greatest joy, but also her greatest challenge. I am sure most of us can relate to that sentiment.

Helen had a singleton vaginal birth with her first child, in which she suffered a bad tear that was 'unrepairable' because of the swelling. She also suffered with shock from the trauma of the birth, which led to her oestrogen levels plummeting much further than they should. Helen experienced extreme fatigue and was repeatedly diagnosed with exhaustion by her GP. After suspecting perimenopause, Helen eventually had a diagnosis of low oestrogen due to the birth trauma: 'my body apparently recoiled so much from the experience that it tried to go into the menopause and stopped producing oestrogen.' As a result, Helen was prescribed topical oestrogen. When I asked Dr Eloise Elphinstone, a UK GP, whether oestrogen is routinely prescribed for postnatal women who have experienced similar symptoms to Helen, she said 'Sometimes topical oestrogen might be prescribed for vaginal dryness postpartum, but systemic HRT (which can be used to help with fatigue associated with menopause, alongside other menopausal symptoms) would not be prescribed. This is an interesting area to explore but the studies are not there yet.'

Helen's second birth came after two months of bed rest due to carrying two full-size babies within her very slight frame. She had a planned abdominal birth, the recovery from which she found difficult due to 'phenomenal pain'. Helen experienced a deep diastasis recti from carrying the twins, which she believes led to an umbilical hernia. A postpartum umbilical hernia is when your intestines start to poke out of your weakened tummy muscles. Helen described it as 'looking like I had a finger poking out above my belly button' and she experienced difficulties with mobility and pain. In a very efficient manner, Helen had surgery to correct this and finally do a proper repair on her perineal tear. When I asked Helen why she elected to have these surgeries at the same time, it was clear that it was the only way she could imagine getting it done at all. There was no way she could spare two rounds of healing time. And this is the truth of our existence as modern mothers when we're juggling all the balls. Taking time out can often be that one piece of the Jenga (other wooden stacking games are available) tower that leads to all the others crashing down. As a mum of three, with a very demanding job, I got the impression that Helen's surgery and healing were part of a lengthy To Do list in a very busy life. She recovered well though, crediting walking to slowly build up fitness again, and voice work to reconnect to her diaphragm, and currently has no issues from either injury.

When discussing her postpartum journey, Helen also sounded apologetic about not knowing the fine detail of her injuries/conditions and her reluctance to 'root around' her nether regions to practise the scar tissue manipulation that her women's health physio had advised. Like so many women, she had done her own research to find out about a women's health physio, and had then shoe-horned the sessions into a jam-packed diary. Homework at this point, especially if it involves sticking your fingers inside yourself to try feel something that you have zero clue about, can be a task too many for us time-strapped mothers. Although we are beginning to feel more comfortable with talking about our bodies, and the roller-coaster of being a woman, many of us are not familiar enough with our most intimate bits to know what is normal and what is not. Helen also pointed out that this kind of touch was nothing like masturbation and was not something she felt comfortable with. We discussed the 'wand' that other women in this chapter have endorsed and I could tell Helen was quite tickled by the magical connotations this conjured up (come on, what other phrase was I going to use?) as well as intrigued as to whether it could help her.

Almost a year on from surgery, Helen is cautious about lifting so as not to undo her hernia repair. She does paddle-boarding to shore up her core strength, and she built a community around her to help support her during her postpartum period, which she describes as 'a hard and lonely time'. When written like this it seems like Helen has done more than enough to navigate her postpartum journey and restore her health, but I got the distinct impression when I spoke to her that she thought she could be doing more. I felt she was being a bit hard on herself – I'm sure we *all* feel we could do more. She stated she could do with doing some Pilates, if she could find the time. She has the intention to build her strength back up to do weights again at the gym and she would love to get to the bottom of her bone-crushing fatigue, but right now, she is doing enough to function, work, be a present mother and experience the joy that being a part of a family of five has brought her.

### Natasha Pearlman

I met Natasha when we were lobbying MPs to influence policy changes in postnatal care. Natasha, then the editor of *Grazia* magazine in the UK, had recently penned an article in *The Times* about her traumatic childbirth experience and was keen to help push for changes that could help women be more informed antenatally and better cared for postnatally.

Natasha describes the birth of her first daughter as, 'horrendous'. She had felt abandoned, in a windowless room, and pushed to her limit to deliver her baby 'naturally' even though she was large, she was back to back, and she was stuck. A challenging 33-hour labour culminated in a difficult pushing stage followed by an episiotomy and forceful forceps delivery. Natasha tells me that she felt physically and psychologically 'destroyed' after this experience. She had to wear huge incontinence pads for the blood, as maternity pads weren't cutting it. She was so swollen that she could not recognise herself and could not even fit into any of her maternity clothes. She was in pain for months afterwards, needing to use an inflatable cushion to sit on for least four weeks postpartum. This, coupled with leaking urine, felt humiliating for Natasha. The psychological fall-out was also considerable: she was constantly shaking and found the smallest tasks difficult to complete. After having walked from her home to the local train station in London for most of her life, this became a personal Everest for her and resulted in her suffering with panic attacks.

When we talk (from her parents' home in London, as she was visiting from New York) she sounds light and breezy and as if this hellish period has been firmly consigned to history. With such a sunny outlook, I was surprised to hear that she was still experiencing symptoms from an anterior and posterior prolapse that happened during her first birth. She told me that sex can be painful still and that she cannot run or do very high intensity exercise as she will leak. I quickly realised that Natasha has found acceptance of her new body and has adapted her lifestyle and exercise regime to ensure that she can remain fit and happy, while not exacerbating any issues. Natasha now does yoga, peloton (training on a static bike) and weight training and has found a great personal trainer who has taught her to utilise and strengthen her pelvic floor while exercising. Natasha has found this incredibly useful, as regular pelvic floor exercises (Kegels) were not featuring in her day-to-day life due to the demanding nature of her job and lifestyle. I was pleased to be able to discuss this, as – for as much as I bang on about doing your pelvic floor squeezes/lifts – it just doesn't work for all people. For whatever reason, if you find you cannot commit to this daily practice, instead of giving up on your pelvic floor you can find other ways to 'train' it – whether that be through Pilates or yoga, or finding a personal trainer who understands pelvic issues. My biggest take-away from our chat was that you have to find a way to stay fit and healthy that works for you and that you will be able to commit to, because if doing something becomes a chore, you will find ways to avoid it and you'll probably end up feeling guilty for not doing it – and this is not what we want.

Natasha also spoke beautifully about how healing her second birth experience was. She had been very open about not wanting a second vaginal birth, and even wondered if she could go through another pregnancy and birth after the trauma of her first experience. She has not been able to request, let alone look at, the notes from her first birth. She had been so deeply bruised by what happened that she found every visit to the hospital and every midwife visit during her second pregnancy difficult and emotional. The difference, she says, this time, was that she felt everyone was on her side. Her choice to have a planned caesarean section was not questioned and she felt supported the whole way. Despite being left until last in the day, the day her second daughter arrived, and despite it being hot and sticky, as it was the middle of a heatwave – Natasha feels wholly positive about the caesarean birth. The way she describes it, it seems it was truly 'woman-centred' with

Natasha being able to help indicate where the incision would go, so as to be hidden afterwards, as well as them creating a very calming environment as she was understandably very anxious. They also did not insist on Natasha holding the baby straight away while she was sewn up, as this was against her wishes. While I know that many people do want to hold their baby straight away, and some are traumatised when they can't, I found this pretty heart-warming. It shows they were really listening to Natasha and respecting her views, feelings and decisions. If I am honest, this is something I don't come across nearly often enough. Natasha summed it up when she said she felt 'heard' – something that was severely lacking in her first birth.

Natasha clearly not only felt in control of her birth, but also her postpartum period. Because she had been through it before, and knew what to expect, she had planned in advance to have help. She chose not to breastfeed and found that this also helped her recovery, as she was able to rest more (she gives a shout out to her husband for doing the night feeds) and find some structure. She gave herself permission to rest more, to have an hour a day to herself, and to allocate time for healing (she saw a postnatal physio who helped with a small diastasis recti). Natasha says 'It wasn't a dream, Thea had allergies, it was still tiring... but it wasn't traumatising.' She deeply wishes other women could be properly educated about what childbirth and postpartum can be like, so they don't feel as ambushed by the whole experience as she did. Reflecting, she says she wishes she had had a doula the first time around as she feels it is really critical, in the system and environment we currently have for birthing women and people in this country, to have someone with significant knowledge and experience who truly has women's best interests at heart, to advocate for you.

Before we ended our call, we discussed, briefly, whether Natasha would consider surgery for the ongoing prolapse issues. I got the impression that Natasha felt it did not significantly negatively impact her life enough for her to consider it right now. She was keen to visit a women's health physio State-side to see if conservative treatment over there might be different and yield more sustainable results. It was 'never say never' on the surgery option, but I could tell she would really want to do her research and be very confident that it would not cause more issues than it was fixing (as has been the case with the mesh scandal, which has left many women disabled across the world). I left Natasha to go off on a family camping adventure, while simultaneously being at the helm of *Glamour* magazine in New York, and I could tell she was a changed woman. Yes, changed by her traumatic entry to motherhood, but also by her resilience, her healing second birth and her acceptance of herself. She tells me she will report back on women's physio USA-style, so watch this space.

### Claire Black

Claire Black, an ex-lawyer and now 'Chief Parent at Home' with two young children, first came to my attention on Instagram. I kept seeing this unassuming looking woman, with a noticeable diastasis recti (she is often in sports gear) doing the most incredible workouts. But, but, but my brain would splutter… should she be *doing that?!* Turns out, yes! And not only should she be doing that, but by showing other people all over the world what can be achieved with regards to postpartum healing, recovery and fitness, she will be creating such a positive ripple effect. I feel so much better informed having only had an hour's call with Claire and I am glad that she seems to be changing the narrative about what is possible if your tummy muscles split.

As we've seen, almost everyone who has a full-term pregnancy will have a degree of diastasis recti. Claire's was quite extreme. She was unaware of it for most of her first pregnancy, until a locum midwife told her to be careful getting off the bed as 'there's a split in your rectus sheath' and then no more was made of it. It wasn't until Claire was at home post-birth and a midwife 'felt all the way down to my bowel' that she was aware there was a problem. As with most new mothers, it wasn't something Claire could focus on as she got to grips with life with a newborn and some pretty awful bouts of mastitis. In fact, her mastitis was so bad that she was referred to a breast clinic. With her focus away from her tummy, it wasn't until she was crawling up the stairs, due to excruciating back pain, that she recognised that something was really awry. Lying in the bath, she began to worry as her tummy was so large and lax that it would ripple with the movement of the water. None of her peers were having the same issue and she knew she still looked heavily pregnant. This was socially isolating as she didn't feel comfortable meeting up with other new mums, who's bodies seemed to be returning to their pre-pregnancy shape with more ease.

Claire went to her GP but felt dismissed. Eventually she requested a referral to a women's health physio and at eight months postpartum, an ultrasound showed that her tummy gap was 8.5cm. Claire suspects that it probably started out at about 11cm, as she had already started working with her physio by the time she had the ultrasound. Claire was lucky in the sense that the diastasis didn't prove debilitating or cause any other obvious pelvic issues, but it did make her feel self-conscious, as people would often ask her when she was due (seriously, why do people do this?! Just stop!) and she needed to continue to wear maternity clothes for a while.

Through her GP's referral, Claire worked with a local physio, Lyndsey Whitson, to help shorten the gap and build core strength. What I found most interesting, and inspiring, about Claire's story was that when she and her physio reached a plateau in her progress, they both did more research and came up with a new plan. This involved teaming up with experts in diastasis recti from other parts of the world. Essentially, they formed a training 'team' that spanned the NHS and private practice – with one physio in Scotland (NHS), one in Northern Ireland and one in Australia. Together, with immense commitment from Claire, they set about a new healing journey that built on what Claire and her NHS physio had already achieved. With this expert input (via the video conference calls that we have all become so accustomed to during the Covid-19 pandemic) from Grainne Donnelly and Anthony Lo, including increased load-bearing exercises such as 'deadbugs' and kettlebell swings,* Claire began to see more progress. Her diastasis shrank to 4.5cm and she was also able to do chin-ups, press-ups and sit-ups. Indeed, she told me that physically she is now able to achieve more than she could pre-pregnancy. Although aesthetics were less of a concern for Claire than functionality, she was pleased to be able to see, week on week, how much flatter her stomach was becoming.

Claire went on to have another baby and is now (at the time of writing) three months postpartum. She found the beginning of the

---

* This type of exercise should only be done under expert supervision and guidance if you have a significant diastasis. Claire also explained that the physios coached her in rotational movements using her torso, as this can become limited in people with DRA.

pregnancy quite anxiety-inducing as she had to dramatically scale back her rehab and her bump appeared very early on. She also became worried that she would not be able to give birth vaginally as her midwife was intimating that the baby would not be able to get into the right position due to Claire's diastasis recti. However, Claire says 'I'm living proof that you can give birth vaginally with diastasis recti. At 37 weeks my baby was head down and when she was born two weeks later, my whole labour lasted 2 hours 52 minutes and the pushing stage was just 13 minutes (she was almost born in the hospital car park!) so to anyone who has read or been told that they won't be able to have a vaginal delivery, or their baby won't be in the right position because of their diastasis recti, that is another myth.' Claire kept strong and fit throughout her second pregnancy, continuing to work with her physio team, which has paid dividends in this recovery. She is also a big advocate for 'belly breathing' and really making sure you are taught how to breathe properly. Claire's advice for other mothers with similar issues is: do not panic, as everyone has a degree of diastasis recti, and everyone will have different gap sizes, depths and functionality (indeed you can have a large-ish gap and still be more functional than someone with a smaller gap as it is more to do with the tension that the abdominal muscles are capable of). She also says not to fear movement. You *have* to move when you have a baby – there is so much lifting and turning involved – and it is not only good for your physical health to move about, it is also good for your mental health. You do need to make sure you are moving correctly and engaging your breath as much as possible. Claire is keen to point out that not moving can cause muscles to atrophy and get weaker, and this really resonated with me. Through becoming so engrossed in 'preserving myself' postpartum, I definitely became afraid to move and it's something that I need to work on even now. I convinced myself I couldn't run or jump, even though I have not (yet) had any cause to think that. And so I stopped. I have definitely become weaker as a result. This is not a klaxon calling you to go ping-ponging around your local trampoline park, but a gentle reminder that you need and deserve to be able to move, not just functionally, but in ways that make you happy or add to your life. And there are ways of getting there.

Claire is fortunate to have had such an understanding and

progressive NHS practitioner who was able to recognise the limitations of her clinical experience (she had never treated anyone with a DRA as severe as Claire's) and collaborate with experts to get the best outcome for her patient. Claire also recognises that she is privileged to have had the time and resources to seek this level of care. Claire is keen to point out to her followers that she works incredibly hard, and with a team, to get the results that she has and that you cannot just jump into the kind of exercises that she is capable of doing now (you should see her chin-up game. Outstanding). She is now 'paying it forward' by chronicling her postpartum recovery on Instagram and speaking with me and on other women's health forums. Her training has got her to a point where she is at peak physical fitness, but she now needs to discuss surgery as, aesthetically, her belly is not shrinking enough for her to feel comfortable. I know she will provide a source of comfort and inspiration for many mothers who are battling with separated tummy muscles.

In her blog, Claire is candid about the emotional and psychological impact of having a DRA. While her confidence in her progress and her strength is obvious, there is a flipside: she still finds social situations difficult as people can still assume she is pregnant. She also struggles to find comfortable clothing. She has found solace in speaking out about this and being contacted by other women who are experiencing the same. She also has a real fear that the 'high impact' training she does may cause pelvic organ prolapse, but she monitors this situation carefully and is not afraid to be seen by a healthcare professional promptly if anything is not feeling right. This is why Claire is passionate about saying that while you can work towards the body you want and improve your strength, you must do so alongside experts who can guide you and help you set your own personal goals and limits.

## ADVICE

I seriously contemplated getting one of those baby-grows for my firstborn that reads 'My Mum Doesn't Want Your Advice'. As a first-time mum, or, indeed, at any time once you are a parent, you will be subject to *a lot* of unsolicited advice about child-rearing. While it is (mostly) given with the best of intentions, it can be a minefield and as a general rule of thumb I suggest people should wait to be asked before imparting their wisdom on everything from how many layers a child should be wearing, to when and how to wean. However, advice on how to have a softer landing on Planet Mother tends to be a bit thinner on the ground and can sometimes be delivered in cryptic puzzles or furtive whispers. Here, 10 mothers shout out some advice to you so that it's loud and clear.

'If you're having a c-section, make sure you have a tonne of pillows around you to help with getting in and out of bed for the first week or so, because that sh*t hurts.' *Stef*

'Get a water cup with a lid and a bendy straw, I found drinking bottles a nightmare because I couldn't tip my head back.' *Lynette*

'Breast shells! Even if you have no intention of keeping your milk. They have a hard plastic outer and a silicone inner with a hole for your nipple. This means nothing whatsoever is touching your extremely bitten-off and sensitive nipples. I called them my bionic boobs. They are also useful if you end up like a drowned rat each time you feed as the other side gets jealous and starts to squirt like crazy.' *Emma and Karina*

'Open and check things as soon as you can, so you are not trying to read instructions with a crying baby. Flashbacks to not putting all the bits back together correctly and pouring formula all over the baby's face when he was screaming.' *Anna*

'When half-asleep don't use the wrong power cable for your expressing machine! A higher voltage plug is not a good idea. It expressed at twice the speed. Not at all comfortable!' *Melissa*

'Baby food pouches – the squeezy fruit and vegetable ones. For you! Great for water intake, a touch of energy, to help you poo and they're easy to grab one-handed.' *Shevi*

A nice cheap jade face roller is perfect for rollering sore blocked milk ducts. *Yolanda*

'Sleep on towels under the bed sheets after giving birth. You will sweat off all the excess fluid you have been carrying around! Makes for very soggy sheets.' *Penina*

# CHAPTER 9

# YOUR PLAN FOR OPTIMAL LONG-TERM HEALTH

If you work in postnatal health, or have an interest in the subject, you may often hear the refrain 'once postnatal, always postnatal'. This is absolutely the case, which is why I think it is so crucial that we see it as an ongoing project to get ourselves to optimal health – and then maintain it. 'Project Me', as it were. There are issues that may surfacce long after the six-week, fourth trimester or one year 'markers'. Some issues may have been underlying before or during pregnancy and some may have been caused by the pregnancy or birth itself.

## THE QUANDARY

Several times in this book I, and others, have implored you to both advocate for yourself and also to try to not do things alone. This is the catch-22 of modern motherhood in the West. We have many *good things*. Huge advances in maternal safety, formula if you need/want it, breastfeeding peer support groups, fluffy pillows and warm houses and microwaves. But there is a lot lacking. In the book we are asking you to simultaneously accept help and reach out for it, and sometimes you will, almost literally, be grasping at straws. Because we are not yet set up properly for nurturing new mothers in the way they need. This is something we seem to have lost along the way to becoming 'civilised'. The reasons for this are cultural, systemic and not easy to unpick. The hospital system for childbirth is not geared toward being woman-centred, and while there are activists both within and outside of the system, creating change, we are still a long way off.

Women don't currently receive consistent holistic support to adapt to new motherhood and recover mind, body and soul. You likely won't see the same midwife or health visitor consistently,* you may miss appointments because they call while you are out or you cannot get to the appointment on time, your GP maternal check may be rushed and limited in scope. When you are discharged you may feel abandoned and still in pieces. And we are asking you to get out there and push for self-care but, simultaneously, rest, recuperate and not do it all yourself. It's a quandary. It's too much. I understand that.

And so, here is my cheat sheet for addressing this quandary:

## 1. TO BE AN ADVOCATE FOR YOURSELF

- In hospital, flag anything that doesn't seem or feel right. You can refuse to leave until you feel well and ready. Ask for a copy of your notes.
- Schedule a GP appointment earlier than 6–8 weeks if you feel you need to speak to someone other than a midwife/health visitor.
- Request a different midwife or health visitor if you do not feel they are helping you.
- Make a note of all your symptoms and track them so that you have the information to hand, even when in a sleep-deprived blur.
- Screenshot our GP prompts from page 50 to take with you to your GP maternal check appointment.
- If, at any point, you feel that your GP or consultant is not listening to, or addressing, your concerns, request to see someone else. Keep going until you find someone who you feel understands you and your problems. You can ask the practice manager if there is anyone with a specialism or interest in perinatal health.
- Push for a referral for a women's health physio. There is meant to be an easy pathway for women from GP to women's health physio on the NHS, but in reality, you can sometimes hit an obstacle. You are entitled to this referral.
- Ask about options in all cases. You can use the **BRAIN** acronym that you may be familiar with from pregnancy, in regards to discussing childbirth options.

   **B – Benefits.** What are the benefits of this option?

   **R – Risks.** What are the risks of this option? You can ask about

* The Maternity Transformation Programme is implementing a 'continuity of care' policy, where this should be rectified within the next decade.

the absolute risk vs the relative risk. This compares the risk for the general population to what the risk is for you, with your individual circumstances. It can also be helpful to ask for numbers to back things up (i.e. a 1 in 100 chance of adverse outcomes). Risk calculations can be tricky to navigate, with communication on risks between health professionals and lay-people open to interpretation. I have found the summary on the WRISK (a project, in conjunction with BPAS on understanding and improving the communication of risk relating to pregnancy) website[80] very helpful.

**A – Alternatives.** What are the alternative options available?

**I – Intuition.** You know your body better than anyone. Listen to your body and don't worry too much about medical jargon or correct terminology when explaining a problem (although some knowledge of your anatomy will obviously help!)

**N – Nothing.** What happens if you don't do anything? Remember, you can revisit options later.

- If you happen to be reading this in advance of having a baby and you live with a chronic illness or condition, try to schedule an assessment with your consultant two to three months postpartum.

- If you are living with a chronic condition/illness, or you are a trans person giving birth, and you want to breastfeed, you can access advice on what medication is suitable for using while lactating on the Drugs and Lactation database (LactMed). This goes for medication you take for mental health issues such as depression, anxiety and psychosis too. The NHS website states that very few medications are unsafe while breastfeeding/chestfeeding, and your healthcare provider should clearly outline the risks and benefits of continuing or starting to take medication.

- If you are in NICU, ask if a midwife can come up and assess you near to where you are, rather than having you limp down to a ward full of mothers holding their babies.

- If you have gone through pregnancy or baby loss, ask if there is a dedicated midwife who helps mothers not only come to terms with loss, but also does your physical checks and assessments.

- If you have experienced sexual trauma in your life, ask if there is someone with specialist trauma training to help you and also do your physical checks and assessments.

## 2. TO BE NURTURED

- Say *yes* to every bit of help. Sometimes that offer only comes around once. Take it. It's hard, I know it's hard. We've been conditioned to try and do it all ourselves and we may feel 'weak' for accepting that offer of a school pick-up for the older kids, or someone stood at our grubby kitchen sink washing up. People want to help, they don't always know how… so just say *yes*.

- Stay in bed. Nothing says 'I need rest' like just refusing to get out of bed. As an added benefit, lying in bed for weeks with your newborn (this is probably only possible with your first) will facilitate bonding and also help with breastfeeding.

- Stay in your pyjamas. A clear, visual indication that you are not 'up to it' yet… whatever 'it' might be.

- This is one for the brave souls who are reading this pre-baby: have a 'mother blessing' instead of a 'baby shower'. A baby shower tends to put all the focus on the baby, with things like gender reveals, cakes depicting cots and all manner of other things (don't Google them <shudders>), and gifts of clothes and teddies for the baby. A 'motherway/blessingway' or 'mother blessing' puts *you* front and centre and is a gentle nudge that you (also) need nurturing by those around you. In case you ask, yes I had a mother blessing. And, although I specified no gifts (because I didn't want to seem like a diva) I was brought food, warm socks and Epsom salts. The message was implanted – I matter too. I didn't know anyone else who had done this, and I felt trepidatious doing it, but the women around me made me feel so special that day. I am so glad I did it.

- Ask for help. Yes, this is right back to advocating for yourself again – but until society cottons on to the fact that women don't just spring up out of bed like some sort of Stepford wife/ Disney princess hybrid, ready to 'show off their post-baby-body' and make *you* a cup of frickin' tea, we need to be plain speaking about when we need help. Ideally, your community (whether that be made up of family or friends or both) will create an environment in which you can rest and recover, as well as keep you hydrated, nourished and comfortable. But if they are not doing this, you may need to ask. I formed a WhatsApp group I named 'Squad' (wonder if this will age well?) and added friends from my town, as I don't have family members nearby, so I could post out emergency requests for help. I am not going to lie, it *does* make me feel awkward asking for help. I only feel better when others from the group ask something of me. Nevertheless, it has been such a security blanket. Likewise, you may need to reach out to ask for help from health professionals (see above) as the offers might not be as forthcoming as they should be.

I asked Maria Booker, the Programmes Director at the charity Birthrights, for advice on how to be your own 'patient advocate' within the current system. Below is a list of things you could consider.

- Trust your own instincts about your body. Research online using reputable websites to gauge whether there is something going on that could be treated. And don't be afraid to speak to your GP/ midwife or health visitor.
- Know that you should be respected and listened to. A good healthcare practitioner will want to hear if you are experiencing any difficulties. You can request to speak to a senior manager if you feel you are being dismissed. Ask to speak to another healthcare professional if you would prefer.
- You can contact PALS (Patient Advice and Liaison Service) at any point to aid you with your advocacy, even if you are still on the postnatal ward. No department likes to 'end up' in PALS.
- It may help to use assertive language rather than asking the healthcare practitioner's thoughts. For example, 'I feel this is not right and I would like this issue addressed.'
- Write down your questions in advance of meeting with the healthcare provider and also write down what you want the outcome of the consultation to be, so that you can ensure your needs have been met before you leave.
- If a practitioner uses jargon ask for a plain English explanation. And take someone with you if you are nervous, as they may be able to help you remember what was said.
- New guidance from the GMC (General Medical Council) says that you can record consultations with medics, which can help you if you forget details or need to listen back when you feel more

relaxed. It is common courtesy, and helps to build trust, to inform the doctor that you want to record the consultation, and why.

I also spoke to my friend Claire Barlow, co-founder of Maternal Pituitary Support, who after advocating for herself within a difficult system, recently had a diagnosis of Sheehan's syndrome (a rare postnatal condition). She says, 'Take your health into your hands. If you are banging the drum, making a noise, and no one is listening, then I strongly recommend a Medichecks women's blood test. Take the results to your GP. Be assertive and clear about what you need. The more I have learnt about my condition, the more I am able to use correct medical language. I have found that I get taken more seriously when I do this.'

When I spoke to Dr Rebecca Moore, a consultant psychiatrist who helps mothers through the perinatal period, we discussed how 'reaching out' and 'advocating for yourself' might simply be too much for some women, for a variety of reasons. And if women *are* reaching out but are met with limited or unhelpful responses, it can almost make matters worse. This is why, alongside changes within our health system, a societal shift needs to happen. We need to ensure that, once we are out of the woods ourselves, we 'reach back' to new mothers and offer our support. The onus cannot be entirely on a new mother, with all of the upheaval that matrescence entails, to seek support: support should also seek her.

Right, so we've addressed the foundations: a need to reach out and also accept help when it is offered. What else?

## CAN YOU HIRE A DOULA?

Doulas are amazing but they are not free (unfortunately we haven't yet caught up with countries like Holland and Germany, which provide much more nurturing for mums in the early days), although, as I mentioned before, the Doula UK organisation does have a 'Doula Access Fund' for those who would struggle to meet the cost themselves. Doula UK describe the role of a doula as someone who 'supports the whole family to have a positive experience of pregnancy, birth and the early weeks with a new baby'. In the UK, doulas are often trained by the Doula UK accredited organisation, but there are also independent trainers, like Mars Lord who runs Abuela Doulas, which has a focus on bringing cultural heritage to the practice of being a 'birth worker'.

A doula is a non-medical birth worker, but they can also help enormously in the postpartum period. As well as being a hands-on help through pregnancy and birth (with research showing they can help reduce medical interventions and enhance birth satisfaction), these women will come to your home to help you adjust to new motherhood and help you with practical jobs (cooking, cleaning, laundry etc) in the house. This can be especially beneficial if you have had a difficult birth or caesarean, you are a single parent or if you already have children. Studies have also shown that having a doula in the postpartum period can increase your chances of establishing breastfeeding,[81] if that's your choice. Hannah Russell, a marketing consultant from Surrey, says 'Having no family nearby, I bit the bullet and arranged for a doula to come and help; it's honestly the best thing I could have done. She did everything and anything from cooking meals and making sure I remembered to eat, to entertaining my older children. I think we sometimes get trapped in that feeling of needing to do it all, when actually we're just putting ourselves under unnecessary pressure.'

I spoke to doula Laura Rice, who trained with Abuela Doulas. She explained just how varied her role is. As well as providing a wonderful postpartum menu (see Chapter 2) for clients to choose from, she helps with laundry, cleaning, school runs and batch cooking, but she also provides 'body work' like Indian head massage. Can you imagine anything more divine, when you are exhausted and giving everything to someone else – than to be nurtured in this way? It almost made me well up when Laura described how she looks after new mothers. In addition to this, she also provides a listening ear for women's worries or helps them work through the emotions attached to the birth experience: 'we sit and chat and I witness what she has been through with no judgement or agenda.'

Laura also explained how having a doula can be particularly reassuring for women and birthing people from black and other minority ethnic backgrounds. With health outcomes in maternity still much poorer for women from these communities (as evidenced in the MBRRACE reports), anything that can make women feel safer in a medical environment is a plus, and having an advocate can make such a difference. A 2013 study showed that women from socially disadvantaged backgrounds fare better with doulas,[82] with less instance of birth-related complications and higher breastfeeding success rates. A 2017 Cochrane review of 26 studies (across 17 countries and involving over 15,000 women) showed that continuous support throughout labour, such as that provided by a doula, can lead to more positive outcomes and more birth satisfaction. Doulas can also help women to express their cultural needs, particularly if there is a language barrier. Laura also spoke to me about the importance of lineage when it comes to birth and postpartum. Doulas can help women, and birthing people, to connect to their own cultural traditions, by identifying together ways they can feel more in touch with their roots. For instance, a doula friend of Laura's learnt some traditional Chinese healing recipes for a client so that she could have these immediately postpartum.

It is also suggested that doulas can help much younger (adolescent) mothers.[83] Also, although there doesn't appear to be data to support this (yet!) it appears that doula support could also be particularly helpful for women and birthing people from other marginalised or underserved communities, such as transgender people, people on the autistic spectrum and those from traveller communities. It stands to reason that if birth workers such as doulas have been proven to improve outcomes for women from some marginalised communities, that this skillset and experience will help them to help others in other similar, albeit disparate, circumstances. However, there are different nuances to consider, so do not assume that every doula will have the same skillset. There seems to be a movement toward a more 'intersectional' approach to midwifery, doula and birth worker work, led in no small part by Mars Lord and AJ Silver of the Queer Birth Club, which accounts for every individual and their unique circumstances. When doing your research, look for someone who represents or speaks positively about your community, has trained with someone who focuses on marginalised communities, or has extensive experience in this area. Beyond that, and speaking from experience, plump for someone you 'gel' with. This person will be with you at your most vulnerable, and in an incredibly intimate set-up it is paramount that you feel comfortable with, and have confidence in, this person.

There is very little negative I can say about the work that doulas do – it seems like such a simple and common-sense addition to perinatal care. It may feel like a luxury, but try to remember that we are simply trying to rebuild the village structure that we lived with for so long, and still need.

## DON'T FORGET YOUR PARTNER

My (long-suffering) husband gamely read this chapter for me in draft form and he pointed out that I have not given nearly enough airtime to dads. This is a totally fair point. The dads (and partners and wives) can do, and often do do (aga-doo-doo-doo) a lot of the heavy lifting (literally and metaphorically) in the early days postpartum. I know some don't, and I know some people manage all of it without partners. But for those with a life partner, if ever there was a time to lean on them, it is now. I firmly believe that my husband's support not only saved me from the clutches of postnatal depression after my first child, but was also the crucial factor in me succeeding in *eventually* establishing breastfeeding. Not only that, he also took the midwife at her word when she said he should 'feed me up' and made me the most exquisite (and obscenely calorific) hot chocolate on demand for weeks. It took me a while to get the recipe out of him, but it turns out that a hot chocolate made with both cream *and* ice cream can really hit that postpartum spot.

We went without a postnatal doula both times, for various reasons, but my husband was more than up to the job of taking care of me. And your partner could be too. With male partners, we could be forgiven for underestimating them, as society likes to perpetuate the trope that they are useless, cannot infer needs and will need constant instruction. While it is true that some men might take a little while to adjust and find their feet, and gentle prompts might be necessary – give them a chance to impress you with *their* caregiving skills. This extends to caring for the baby too. It's not all on you. Some men will take to this like veritable ducks to water. In same-sex couples, the dynamic might be a little different, and it is said that the 'domestic load' is more evenly split between married/co-habiting women in the first place, so the adjustment *may* not be so great. But, of course, not everyone fits any given stereotypical mode, and we all need to find our feet. Try to play to each other's strengths to make a formidable team. I am not going to pretend this is easy. It isn't. But, if you have a partner, then *use them*. They should be in absolute awe of the feat you have just carried out and a naughty hot chocolate and a foot rub should be the least you can expect.

## TRUST YOUR INSTINCTS

You will be told numerous times to trust your instincts as a mother. You can also use this superpower for yourself. You know your body. You know what feels right and what feels wrong, and you will often have an instinct about why. There are huge gaps in research in women's health, and if you are not getting the response you need from your healthcare team, then do your own research. I remember an obstetrician-gynaecologist asking me, with a sneer, if I had done my research on Mumsnet when talking about birth options. Apart from the fact I had actually spread my research far and wide, including using PubMed, I was riled that he was so quick to discount what is essentially a huge pool of female experience. With the advent of the internet, women can communicate and find mirrors to our own experiences. We are filling in the gaps left by the lack of research. While I have the utmost respect for evidence-based principles, where evidence is based on robust trials, I hold no truck with dismissing thousands and thousands of accounts from women of the same symptoms as 'anecdotal'. So, if you're feeling something isn't right, and other women are echoing this back to you, feel confident about getting it addressed. We've spent too long being told things are all in our heads, or we are 'hysterical' – when, in fact, modern medicine treats the male as 'the norm' and us as 'the other' and we are *still* regularly misunderstood.* You know you. Our sisters know their bodies. Listen to your body and listen to other women. This view was reflected back to me by obstetrician-gynaecologist Dr Sunita Sharma, who said, 'In postnatal care, there are very few high-quality research papers

---

* For further reading on this topic, do check out Caroline Criado-Perez's book *Invisible Women*.

and this limits the strength of NICE recommendations in this field. However, no evidence doesn't mean that symptoms don't exist or don't need to be addressed.' Exactly that.

## GO AND SEE YOUR GP

Dr Eloise Elphinstone says that you can go to your GP, at any point, with a complaint or issue that relates to pregnancy and birth – no matter how many weeks, or even years, after the event. She also gives brilliant advice on how to approach embarrassing issues. The following has been taken (with permission) from Eloise's Instagram account (in partnership with the MASIC Foundation):

- Remember, as doctors we see all sorts of things, so nothing tends to phase us and we don't get embarrassed.
- Everything that is told to us is strictly confidential, nothing leaves the consultation room, other than if we need to do a referral and we will ask your permission.
- A lot of women are in exactly the same position as you, you are not alone. Therefore, as GPs, we have talked to a lot of women about similar issues.
- Try to see a doctor who you know, and you feel comfortable with.
- Book a double appointment, if possible, to give you time to talk.
- Try not to wait to see your GP for something else, or wait until your six-week check. You need allocated time to focus on this one problem.
- If you are nervous, tell your doctor. Hopefully they can put you at ease.
- If you don't feel comfortable talking about it, some GP practices now have the ability to send an online query.
- Try to be as direct as possible – tell the doctor exactly what is worrying you.
- Don't worry if you don't know the right term, just explain it as best you can.
- If possible, try to go to your appointment on your own, without any children or interruptions, it makes it easier for you to concentrate and your GP focus on you.
- Take a list of questions with you. It means you won't forget to ask

anything and also can help asking embarrassing questions, as you are reading off your paper.

- It can be helpful to take a diary of your symptoms/feelings to show your GP.
- Ultimately, as GPs – we are here to help, and we really want to help. If you don't think we have understood, please tell us.

## GO AND SEE A WOMEN'S HEALTH PHYSIO

Have I mentioned this before?! I jest. I know I have harped on about this a lot, but as the featured case studies show, these practitioners really are able to address and rectify a wide range of significant health issues and, if not, they will be best placed to help you prepare your body for any surgery you may need. I have tried to go for a check-up, not only after my births, but annually. I have seen both NHS and private practitioners and have found each one incredibly knowledgeable, sensitive and reassuring. This is what you can, generally, expect from your appointment:

- You will sit down and go through your health history, including your births.
- They will ask you if you are suffering with any pain, discomfort, issues with sex or continence issues (Edel says patients generally needed to be prompted on continence or sexual issues as they don't offer this information themselves, out of embarrassment. Rest assured, a women's physio has seen and heard it *all* – they specialise in pee, poo and sexual issues).
- They will give you privacy to remove the bottom half of your clothing (I sometimes wear a dress or skirt, as it somehow feels more comfortable to keep 'something' on!) and lie on the bed, where you will likely drape some blue paper or a clean towel over your lower half. They will ask when they can come back in.
- They will ask you to part your legs (usually with soles of feet together and knees flopping outwards, although practitioners vary and will make sure you are in a position that is comfortable to you) and, wearing surgical gloves with lube on them (they will ask if you are allergic to either of these), they will insert a finger, or more fingers if comfortable, and begin the assessment.

- The assessment will consist of looking at the tissue of the vagina and assessing if it looks and feels healthy (good colour, lubricated) or is in need of a bit of TLC. They will then feel around the inside of your vagina and 'palpate' (a medical term, which simply means 'touch') the tissue to assess whether there are areas of tightness and scar tissue. They may find points in the tissue which are painful. With your permission, they may do 'trigger point release' whereby they gently press the tissue to allow it to release (it feels a bit like how a masseur would 'release' tension in your shoulder).

- They will then ask you to try lifting/squeezing your pelvic floor muscles (they may use the term 'contract' or they may give you a verbal cue like 'try to hold my finger' or 'pretend your muscles are a lift going up') and this will help them gauge whether you are doing your 'Kegels' correctly. As I mentioned earlier, many women do not know how to properly engage, lift and release their pelvic floor muscles and it is important you do it properly to ensure you are benefitting and not making any issues worse.

- Your practitioner will be able to tell if you have any degree of prolapse. If they are very thorough, they may have you stand up as well, so that they can do the assessment in standing position, as obviously our anatomy changes from standing to lying (as those who have an interest in active birth will know!). I watched a video of some incredibly diligent women's health physios not only assessing a woman standing, but also assessing her as she did squats and weights. I am not going to lie, the one time I was assessed standing up felt super weird, but I definitely think it is worthwhile and also, it kind of fits with our move towards women being active participants in their own healthcare rather than passively lying down as 'things are done to us'.

- Some practitioners may also ask to assess your rectum, if you had a third/fourth-degree tear or are experiencing faecal incontinence. If you find this too uncomfortable, you can politely decline, but these are experienced and sensitive practitioners, who only value returning you to health.

- Your practitioner may talk you through everything they are feeling and their review as it is happening and others may wait until your sit-down debrief at the end. I prefer a bit of both. They will talk you through whether your pelvic floor is hypotonic (weak) or hypertonic (tight), although it will most likely be a mix of both(!), and what you can do to make it heal and function better. They will talk you through any degree of prolapse. Edel was very reassuring when we spoke, stating that research suggests around 50% of women (over the age of 50) have some degree of prolapse on visual (objective) examination, but many are completely asymptomatic and it does not affect their life (subjectively).[84] If you are having any issues which the prolapse and/or pelvic floor issues are causing, or exacerbating, then the practitioner will work with you to establish a plan to alleviate symptoms and improve pelvic floor function. Edel made a great point when we spoke: 'People's compliance is essential. They have to want it for themselves. You can't do it for them.' Essentially, a practitioner can give you all the tools, but unless you commit to the changes and exercises, it may be fruitless.

- They will likely schedule more appointments to assess improvement. With some cases follow-up may not be needed and with very straightforward cases, there may only need to be one or two maintenance follow-ups. With more severe issues, six or more sessions may be needed. I would highly recommend annual checks, whatever the outcome.

- If any kind of gynaecological assessment makes you anxious or triggers trauma, it is absolutely worth mentioning this to your physio. For example, if you have been the victim of sexual assault, or you have had a traumatic birth or experiences of loss, it is a good idea to flag these. Women's health physios are very gentle (of all the gynae-type exams I have had, I can hand-on-heart say that these have been the most comfortable), but knowing this info will help both of you to ensure a comfortable and well-paced assessment.

If you cannot face an in-person session, then do ask if your physio would do an online consultation. While their assessment will obviously be more limited, the women in this profession are desperate to help you and I am sure they will be happy to accommodate your request.

## GO AND SEE YOUR CONSULTANT

You are not a nuisance. Whether it be a long-term condition that is flaring/needs attention or a new ailment that is impacting your quality of life and/or mental health, you are worthy of having this addressed by a specialist. The NHS is a wonderful health system, manned by fantastic humans, but it is not 'free': we pay taxes (although some would argue not enough to keep it running at the level that it needs to for staff and patients alike!) and you are *entitled* to receive care. In fact, the health service would thank you for getting issues addressed promptly, potentially before they become more serious, as, ultimately, this will likely save money for the service in the long term.

## CONSIDER COUNSELLING

I have heard quite a number of stories of women who only realised with hindsight that they had been suffering with postnatal depression, or another postnatal mood disorder. Yes, you could simply be exhausted, or depleted, or overwhelmed. Or your hormones could be so out of whack, or your adjustment to motherhood so physically assaulting, that this messes with your mind. But it is worth exploring whether it *could* be postnatal depression/anxiety, post-birth PTSD, postpartum psychosis or something else. Again, you are worthy of care. Even if you don't flag up to the healthcare professionals as a case to pursue, after filling in the various mental health surveys after birth, you know *you*. If you are not feeling right – whether one day or one year (or more!) postpartum, let your healthcare provider (likely your GP) know. There is so much more awareness about mental health now, and a growing awareness about the prevalence and wide-ranging effects of birth trauma, that if you reach out, there will be a hand to grab yours. That said, waiting lists can be long, and some medics may not be as sensitive as others, and so we have listed some organisations at the back of this book that you can approach for help. The most prominent would be PANDAS www.pandasfoundation.org.uk.

## CONSIDER COMPLEMENTARY THERAPIES

There are so many complementary/alternative therapies (maybe we should just start calling them therapies now!) available that can help you find your way back to yourself: whether that be realigning your spine to simply making you feel more grounded. Whether you love 'all the woo' or are strictly an 'only the GP and only if absolutely necessary' type, I guarantee that at the very least, an hour to yourself to hear yourself think will feel like a mini-break for your mind, body and soul in the early days. Start gently, with something you're comfortable with, like a massage. A friend of mine bought me a body scrub and massage at a local salon for my birthday present a few months after I had my son. I felt like a new woman afterwards. To have my body touched and nurtured in that way, after spending months doing all the touching and nurturing, was bliss. And the bonus was that my scaly skin was sloughed off and I felt less like a lizard, and more like the woman I was before kids.

Complementary and alternative medicines (often abbreviated to CAM) are recognised as 'a diverse group of health-related therapies and disciplines which are not considered to be a part of mainstream medical care' and include osteopathy, chiropractic therapy, acupuncture, herbal medicine, and homeopathy.[85] Most people seeking these therapies have musculoskeletal or mental health issues they want to address. A survey conducted on this type of care concluded that 12–16% of the population seek CAM therapies. Unsurprisingly, the majority of these people are women from higher socio-economic areas. That said, around 20% of this number are from GP/NHS referrals. This will depend both on the area where you live (postcode lottery, anyone?) and how open and educated your GP is on alternative therapies. I am very lucky that my GP has referred me for both osteopathy (to sort out my pelvic girdle pain) and acupuncture. If you are living with cancer, or another disease or condition, you may find that your GP is more open to referring you to a CAM practitioner. I look forward to a time when medicine more reliably spans both mainstream and alternative therapies and embraces a more holistic approach. In my own experience, alternative therapies have been extremely helpful. My pelvic girdle pain (PGP) was sorted in just one osteopathy session and I have found therapies like herbalism, acupuncture and reiki extremely helpful in healing from my miscarriages.

Most alternative/complementary therapies are not available on the

NHS, so I appreciate that not all women will be able to access them. However, some practitioners *may* offer a 'pay what you can' policy, or similar, to make their particular discipline more accessible, so it is worth enquiring about this.

If you have the means, but are sceptical, you may take heart from the fact that my husband, who works in clinical research (an actual scientist, helping to develop actual drugs) has, when he has been unable to get to the root of physical ailments, acquiesced to my gentle persuasion and tried a few of the therapies mentioned below. I'm not going to say he is now a die-hard holistic therapy fan, or anywhere near it, but he has definitely felt the benefit of treatments that pick up where mainstream medicine sometimes falls a bit short. The more reluctant or trepidatious among us might also like to read this from the NHS website www.nhs.uk/conditions/complementary-and-alternative-medicine.

It is worth noting that not all therapies will suit all people, and, equally, not all practitioners and service-users are a good match. I have definitely had better results with some practitioners over others, even within the same discipline. If you have the time and means to explore some different therapies, until you find one that suits you, then that would be beneficial. I am well aware that this is a privilege and luxury, and so – for the rest of us – I would implore you not to give up after your first try. While one type of therapy might not provide the results you are looking for, another one might really hit the spot.

Disclaimer: if you pursue an alternative therapy, do make sure your practitioner is registered with a relevant body and check with them that there are no contraindications (reasons not to proceed, such as side-effects that you would be susceptible to) to treatment.

**Osteopathy.** According to the General Osteopathic Council, osteopathy is 'a system of diagnosis and treatment for a wide range of medical conditions [...] Osteopaths use touch, physical manipulation, stretching and massage to increase the mobility of joints, to relieve muscle tension, to enhance the blood and nerve supply to tissues, and to help your body's own healing mechanisms. They may also provide advice on posture and exercise to aid recovery, promote health and prevent symptoms recurring'. Osteopath Gemma Dawson adds that there are lots of overlaps with other practices, like physiotherapy and chiropractic practices, but that osteopathy looks at the body as a whole. An important note on cranial osteopathy is that many mothers/ parents find that babies respond very well to it, especially if the birth has been difficult (forceps etc) or if there are problems breastfeeding. Obviously, the more effectively a baby can breastfeed, the less pain or discomfort for you.

Although most people access osteopathy privately, the NHS website states that you can sometimes access this on the NHS, depending on where you live. The first time I went for osteopathy (on the advice of a friend who had become a mother before me), I did not know what to expect. I wondered if there would be some cracking of necks and backs, which I didn't like the sound of, but my practitioner was exceptionally gentle. With cranial osteopathy you may feel like you are just 'lying there' while someone cradles your head or pelvis in their hands. However, they are subtly working with all of your body's systems and I distinctly remember her saying 'I'm just going to move your liver back' (it having been shoved out of place during pregnancy). I was a tiny bit taken aback by this! A few months postpartum she said 'I'm going to move this cough on' and my cough disappeared. I was sold after that. If osteopathy on the NHS isn't available to you, and private care is beyond your budget, then do listen to Ana Mattos, a very experienced family-focused osteopath from Brazil, on the free Postnatal FAQ podcast. One of her recommendations includes warm baths with magnesium for back pain. If nothing else, listen for her beautifully soothing voice!

**Acupuncture.** Don't skip this if you don't like needles! Needle-phobia is a common phenomenon (apparently one in 10 of us is afraid of needles) and your acupuncturist will be very used to helping people to overcome this. Acupuncture treatment involves the insertion of very fine needles into specific points on the body to regulate the flow of 'qi' (pronounced 'chee') along pathways in the body known as meridians. It sounds wacky as hell, but it is rooted in a practice that is 2,500 years old and its efficacy is such that this is one of the CAM therapies most often accessed through NHS referrals. Indeed, I also had acupuncture through a NHS referral. Acupuncture is often used to help treat fertility issues as well as antenatally, but it can also be used in the postpartum period to help the body find equilibrium by calming the nervous system. Studies are, as yet, inconclusive, but there is some evidence that acupuncture can help postnatal depression in some instances.[86] There is also limited research that indicates that acupuncture in the early postpartum period can help with establishing and maintaining breastfeeding.

**Closing the Bones.** This is a ceremony that originated in South America. It is something I would have loved to have indulged in, but I didn't know about it the first time around and didn't have the opportunity the second time around. The methods and experience may vary from practitioner to practitioner, but generally it will involve your hips being tied with, rocked and/or cradled in a 'rebozo' (a special woven cloth, traditionally made by indigenous women from Mexico) and your womb/pelvic area being massaged with warm oils. All of this is with a view to creating good blood flow to the pelvis and closing energy fields which have been opened throughout pregnancy and birth. It is also a celebration of all that your body has achieved. Doula and healer Sophie Messager says, 'it is not only a pleasant massage, it is also a ritual that celebrates and honours the new mother, and can be very healing both physically and emotionally'.

**Mindfulness and meditation.** Saying this is something we can all access for free is the same as saying that breastfeeding is free. It's not really free, as it takes up your time – you may not have much time, or it may take up time when you could be earning (although I am among a growing number of mothers who are doing both). However, it is as free as it can be, notwithstanding the apps and books that might be useful to get you into the swing of it. A mother's time is often considered cheap, but in actual fact, we have very little of it to spare. It really is a precious commodity. I promise that using any window of time you may have to do one of these practices will fill your cup much more satisfyingly than scrolling on your phone or watching *The Real Housewives of Cheshire* (I'm more of a Beverly Hills gal!).

Mindfulness and meditation are not the same thing. As Chopra.com says 'We live in a time when Eastern philosophy is beginning to seep into the mainstream Western way of life. Words like mindfulness and meditation are becoming everyday terms in Western colloquialism, but these words aren't interchangeable'. Mindfulness is the description of being present in the moment and noticing the world around you and how you are experiencing it, including tuning in to your senses. An example of this would be a walk in the park where you notice the wildlife and other people and what movements they are making, what sounds you can hear, what your skin feels like in the breeze and the sound of your footsteps (and maybe a chocolate melting in your mouth… just me?). Meditation is a practice rooted in (usually seated) stillness and breath-work. The aim is to try and clear your busy mind (that ticker-tape that so many of us mothers have on a constant loop) and restore a sense of calm and peace. Using the breath exercises noted in this book, while sitting comfortably, could be a good place to start. If you are able to carve three minutes out one day (I *know* how impossible even this crumb of time can feel) then maybe, over time, you could build this up. Other good resources are the Chopra.com website mentioned above and apps like Calm (Cillian Murphy can lull you to sleep on this one. Sold) and Headspace.

**Reflexology.** Reflexology is a 'touch therapy' with a belief system rooted in a 'map' of the body which corresponds to different areas. Most people will envision all of the attention being directed at your feet, but actually reflexologists may also use gentle pressure on your hands, face and ears as well. I have had reflexology a few times over the years, though not in the perinatal stage, and found it deeply relaxing. A friend, Julia Govan, a mum of two in Edinburgh, credits reflexology with helping her have a more positive, quicker birth the second time around.

**Reiki.** I'm a reiki practitioner myself and I am a big, big fan. It is a form of energy healing that originated in Japan. I find it incredibly soothing. You will find that the practitioner uses their hands to help soothe the body, but it is not a massage. You may experience very warm sensations in parts of your body and even 'see colours'. You can ask your practitioner if they can translate this for you. I had a reiki session after my third miscarriage and I felt a deep release from my throat: it was almost inexplicable. It turns out that the throat and the womb are considered to be 'connected' by many practitioners (I was amazed when I saw images showing how the larynx mirrors the uterus. I have these on my instagram @postnatalhealthcommunity. It also strengthens the whole 'floppy face, floppy fanny' analogy – see page 98).

If this is not something you can afford, an alternative would be to lie somewhere quiet (I know this in itself can be a challenge!) with some reiki music (you can find this on YouTube) playing as you place your cupped hands on different parts of your body and do deep breaths concentrating on the area of the body you are touching – sending that area love. If you have a partner that you trust that can do this for you, this would be just as beneficial, if not even more so. This is great, as being a good masseur/masseuse is not a pre-requisite and cannot be used by your partner as a fob-off! In case the Reiki community get up in arms (unlikely... we tend to be a chilled-out bunch!) I am obviously aware that reiki is more than 'just touch' – in fact, sometimes it's a 'hands-off' treatment – but there is no denying that soothing touch will help kick-start the parasympathetic nervous system and aid relaxation/rejuvenation.

**Herbalism.** Does what it says on the tin, really. Treats (or helps prevent!) issues by using plants/herbs. This treatment, like many of the others, has been used for millennia. In fact, it is the precursor for today's modern mainstream medicine. Indeed, medical herbalism requires an honours degree certification and knowledge of orthodox medicine and diagnostic skills. Some herbs will be immediately familiar, like chamomile. As herbs are generally ingested, it is wise to use a degree of caution and do your research thoroughly on your practitioner and the side-effects of anything they prescribe (particularly as quite a few natural substances can interfere with breastfeeding or other medications).

Other therapies you could explore are: Ayurveda, homeopathy, aromatherapy, naturopathy, Amanae, EMDR (Eye movement desensitization and reprocessing, used for trauma), hypnotherapy, Alexander technique, Bowen technique and Rolfing structural integration, among many, many others. Alternative therapies tend to be 'holistic' in that they do not just treat the physical or mental in isolation, and neither do they tend to focus on one condition/symptom/ailment – but rather the body as a 'whole' system where one thing affects numerous others. In this way, it can be particularly helpful if you are experiencing mood/emotional issues at the same time as physical symptoms. These therapies are often about creating balance in the body, which, in turn, helps create balance in the mind. That said, I would not advocate pursuing alternative/complementary therapies as your first-line or only mode of treatment if you are experiencing moderate to severe physical or mental health issues.

A note on alternative therapies: It is always worth being mindful that some of these practices may originate from countries, cultures or communities that have been ill-served (to put it mildly) by the West in the past. With that in mind, it is worth doing your research on the origins of the practice and its cultural context, with a view to ensuring respect for the complex history which precedes it.

## HYDRATE

I'm gonna say this one last time, and loudly, for those at the back. Drink some bloody water. Drink lots. It helps your energy levels, your blood flow, your hormones, your digestion, your ability to concentrate, your ability to breastfeed, it reduces headaches. Water is life. Drink it with cucumber and mint in it, drink a gallon of fruit tea, drink it cold, drink it warm, drink it however you want to my lovelies – just drink it. This is especially important once you begin to take up more exercise. And did you know that our cycles affect how much water we need? Oestrogen and progesterone affect how water is absorbed, meaning that when these hormone levels drop, water 'leaks' into other tissues (bloating, anyone?) instead of staying in the blood vessels. This can make you feel fatigued, make exercise much harder and also make period cramping worse. In addition, if you are having much heavier periods after childbirth, the excessive blood loss could also leave you feeling dehydrated.

I do not drink as much now I am 18 months postnatal as I did in the early days. And it shows – in my skin, in my energy levels, in my digestion. I might get a neon sign put up in my house to remind me to take my own medicine.

## YOUR PHONE

Mobile phones are brilliant for us mothers. We can access tips and advice at the drop of a hat. We can connect with other parents much more easily. We can work from our phones while at the park with the kids (whether this is furthering a feminist flexi-working cause or kindling flames of burnout is yet to be decided). Phones can provide apps for connecting with other mothers (Peanut, Mush etc), rest (such as Nourish) menstrual tracking (Cycles), and general health and wellness. *But* too much use can also further disrupt our sleep, cause repetitive strain in our poor mum thumbs and create tension in our necks and backs. I'd be Mrs Hypocrite of Hypocrite-Land if I told you to 'use in moderation', as I currently absolutely do not do this. But I intend to. So, there you go. Just something to think about if you're feeling tired, wired and achey. I sometimes find that if I accidentally leave my phone at home for a day, I feel an immense sense of lightness and freedom. One thing that you could consider, which I have utilised on and off, is a 'digital sunset', where you choose a time in the evening when you will physically turn your phone off and leave it in another room overnight. When I remember to do it, I almost feel my body sag with relief. That shows how 'on' we are when we're connected to our phone 24/7. It is also so very tempting to compare your life, house, body, recovery, and offspring with every Trisha, Danni and Henrietta on social media, who sometimes present veritable utopias of motherhood atop a glistening and lithe MumBod. Avoid, avoid, avoid. Two phrases have helped keep that particular green-eyed monster at bay for me: 1. Comparison is the thief of joy. 2. Do not compare their showreel with your 'behind-the scenes'. Also, my own personal mantra: 'It's all bollocks anyway'.

## MOVE ABOUT

As much as I have stressed the need to prioritise rest during your postpartum recovery, lying prone for long periods is not advisable. You need movement to help blood flow and lymphatic drainage. Movement helps healing, digestion and relieves aches and pains, as well helping to release endorphins, which can improve your mood.

You're going to struggle to find a health practitioner that does not advocate moving your body. As with breathing, eating and drinking – it is a fundamental for life. Of course, there are going to be hurdles at some points during your postpartum recovery, and in life in general. I am not suggesting that you dimly attempt to jump over these hurdles. However, a simple reframing might help you. For example, instead of focusing on what you *cannot* do, maybe try focusing on what you *can* do. So, for example, when I was bed-bound after my c-section I could not initially easily walk about as some were encouraging me to do – but I *could* move my feet, legs and arms in bed and I could do my pelvic floor exercises – all of which helped with getting my blood flowing. I could not go to any fitness classes early on in my postpartum period with either son, for various reasons, but I *could* look up a Youtube 'postnatal-friendly' guided session, even if it was only 10 minutes every other day. That, coupled with frequent walks with the baby in the fresh air, really helped me.

Longer term, if you are living with health issues, as a result of pregnancy and birth or otherwise, there may be adaptations that you can make, but it may take perseverance and creativity. For example, a woman with prolapse may be able to run comfortably again if using a pessary, or you might take up something with less impact, such as cycling. Or if you are struggling with fatigue, a sit-down yoga or Tai Ch'i class (probably frequented by older persons; these are our elders – it'd be good to connect with their wisdom) might help you get the blood flowing and boost your mood.

If you're drastically short on time (who isn't these days?) remember that *any* physical activity you do with your children – be it woodland walks, chasing them around a park or a kitchen disco – is exercise. And do heed what Kim Vopni told me about mothers underestimating how much exercise and physical exertion they pack in to one day!

You can see what classes and clubs are available locally for postnatal women. There will often be flyers on notice boards at children's centres, local community centres and in cafes. Osteopath and Pilates instructor Gemma Dawson recommends not only doing your research, to make sure any instructor has undertaken postnatal training, but also trying to look for a small, focused group. She feels it is just as important that you feel comfortable with, and confident in, the instructor.

I remember going down to my local gym, when my firstborn was about six months old. I was desperate both for some time away, and to start regaining some strength, and I was guided through some exercises to do by the instructor at the gym. She wanted me to be doing planks and squats with weights. 'Um, will that affect me if I have a diastasis recti?' I asked gingerly. I must add that I didn't really know what I was talking about but had heard the term. The instructor looked absolutely flummoxed and had no idea what I was talking about. Suffice to say I did not become a gym bunny there (or anywhere actually!). One accreditation that has received widespread acclaim is the 'Holistic Core Restore' programme, which has been developed by personal trainer Jenny Burrell, whom I have heard speak with enthusiasm and deep knowledge about enabling women to recover and thrive.

As you age, bone health should also become a motivating factor. Although women lose bone mass while breastfeeding, they replenish this once the baby has weaned. Unicef asserts that, 'After weaning, lactating women gained significantly more bone in the lumbar spine than did non-lactating women (5.5 versus 1.8%). Earlier resumption of menses was associated with a smaller loss of bone during lactation and a greater increase of bone after weaning.' This is good news for breastfeeding mothers, who often worry about the calcium being 'leached' (nice) from their bones during lactation. That said, we cannot rest on our laurels. Weight-bearing exercise slows bone loss (which can happen as oestrogen is depleted later in life) and actually builds new bone. To avoid osteoporosis, and stay strong, weight-bearing and resistance exercise (think: hiking, light weight work, climbing, dancing) is a must.

## EAT WELL

Again, there's barely been a health expert that I have spoken to who has not stressed that it is important to maintain a healthy weight. And we all know it. We *know* maintaining a healthy weight will likely increase our longevity and decrease our susceptibility to chronic and acute disease. What that weight is depends entirely on you. Size 10 can do one, as being healthy is not a 'one-size-fits-all' solution. BMI (Body Mass Index) is currently used to determine a healthy weight for your height, but has drawn criticism for not painting a clear enough picture of someone's overall health. It doesn't take in to account other factors, such as susceptibility to certain diseases and its measurements, although broadly indicative of overall health, can be wildly 'off' for some individuals. For example, a sportsperson with significant muscle mass may be identified as 'obese' using the BMI method, as it only uses height and weight measurements, and does not discriminate between the weight of fat and the weight of muscle. BMI is predicated on a very old data model that was primarily based on white European men, making it unrepresentative of vast swathes (indeed the 'global majority'!) of people and does not take in to account racial differences, such as South Asian people being more at risk of metabolic disorders (like diabetes) at lower BMI levels than white people, and the differences in body composition between people of different races. On top of that, *where* fat is stored on your body does not feature when looking at BMI as a measure of health and obesity. As mentioned before, it is thought that excess fat around your tummy area is more damaging than fat on your bum or thighs.

Health professionals Professor Debra Bick and Dr Iona Thorne both stressed how being a healthy weight when you become pregnant can decrease your likelihood of developing gestational diabetes or blood pressure-related conditions. Being a healthy weight will also decrease pressure on your pelvic organs, making stress urinary incontinence and pelvic organ prolapse less likely. We're not looking for the much-lauded 'bounce back' into your pre-pregnancy jeans, we're not looking for excess weight loss, and we are certainly not condoning restrictive dieting, or feeling ashamed of your body. This is such a tricky subject, as not only is the postnatal period (and, later on, the perimenopausal period) of your life very vulnerable and a time when you can begin to feel negative about your body, but I am also loathe to focus on weight loss when we are bombarded with images of what we should and *should not* look like from the day dot. I, for one, am heartily sick of *that*. So, while I 100% agree with all of the health professionals I have spoken to, about how important it is for your long-term health to try to maintain a healthy weight, I also want to say 'Go easy on yourself'. It takes a while for the post-birth weight to come off. If you're an 'emotional eater' like me, then life events can throw you off-course when it comes to maintaining healthy habits. And you may be a person who does not fit the mould, who will never be 'slim' in our modern Western understanding of the word, but you may still be very healthy. Journalist Rose Stokes put this perfectly when she said, 'the assumption that bodies larger than society's ideal are automatically seriously unhealthy is outdated and misleading.' Rose is a size 16–18 and is something of a gym addict, regularly swimming, spinning and lifting weights. Indeed, if you are feeling self-conscious about exercising, Rose's articles and social media account will likely provide excellent motivation and reassurance.

Using BMI as the sole indicator of how healthy you are may not be right for you, so try to do some research, and also find health and fitness practitioners who can help you paint a clearer picture for yourself about where your strengths and weaknesses might be. This can involve looking at your family history, measuring your stomach circumference and looking at the areas of your diet that work and those that don't. There is *so* much information out there on diet – what to eat, what not to eat, when to eat it – that it can be very overwhelming. I'd pick a couple of good, evidence-based sources, where the focus is on being healthy rather than dieting or losing weight, and stick to them. The NHS Eat Well information is a good place to start, but it *does* suggest using a BMI calculator, which *may* not be right for you, and it doesn't go into details about food intolerances or alternatives. You could also have a look at Maeve Hanan's book *Your No-Nonsense Guide to Eating Well,* or *Gut* by Giulia Enders, to understand more about what is going on inside.

As someone whose weight fluctuates, I can sympathise with the best intentions not always resulting in the action we need to take. I'm really, really interested in nutrition, and I *know* what I need to eat (and what I need to limit!) to be healthy and the correct weight for my size. I don't always do it though, whether it be because of stress, illness, being distracted, being in social situations where I find it difficult to choose healthy options… the list is long. I have something of a sweet tooth and I love chocolate. When I'm rested and rational, I can incorporate my beloved chocolate and desserts into a broadly healthy diet (as I did when on a strict diabetes diet during pregnancy, which I managed without drugs); but when I am strung out and wrung out, this becomes much more difficult. I definitely have periods where I could treat myself better. Because that's what it is. Eating healthily and exercising is self-care, and it's treating my body with respect. It's investing in how I feel now and my long-term health. There is not one way of eating that is going to suit us all. I abhor diets: they are proven to only work short-term, which is why there is so much so-called yo-yo dieting. As well as being short-term solutions, many diets are too restrictive and do not allow for variety. A restrictive diet may mean you don't ingest the optimum amount of nutrients, and adversely affect your gut microflora (microbiome, which as we've said before is so critical to feeling well and general good health).

You need to find a way to eat healthily that suits you, your body, your family, your culture, your lifestyle, your budget. Broadly speaking, the following may help you: a food diary (for noting how you feel after certain foods, including if you feel sluggish, bloated or have mood changes) and engaging with a GP or other health practitioner if you find you are not tolerating certain foods well, as this could indicate an intolerance. The food diary can also show you clearly what you eat in a day and whether there are emotional or environmental triggers to over-eating or eating foods you'd rather avoid. The other tips I have are:

- Carry healthy snacks for you as well as for your children. If you can eat them, then nuts, seeds and dried fruit can see you through a 'hangry' (when your hunger makes you angry) patch. I often try to eat an apple on the way to school as I know then that I have ingested *one good thing* in my day! I like nuts that taste like a treat so, although they're expensive, I love cashews and macadamia nuts.
- Batch cook. This is something I aspire to rather than something I do. I used to do it and the bliss of reaching for a 'ready meal' that is *actually* a healthful wholesome meal cooked by you (or your partner!) is sweet. It's also really good for economising. Our current lack of freezer space means I can't do this – but it remains a goal.
- Variety: this is good to increase the diversity of your gut flora (and a happy gut equals a happy mind and body) as well as staving off boredom – for you and your family. It's really easy to get stuck in a rut and so I find asking other time-strapped families what they're eating provides me with some new (attainable) inspiration.

- Use baby-weaning recipes. They are *so* easy (those cookery writers *know* how strapped for time we are) and they tend to be healthy and low in salt. I still use a few regularly, including a Thai green curry recipe with white fish that takes 10 minutes.
- Cheat. I am a 'scratch cook' but I am also a cook that regularly has only half the ingredients needed for any given recipe in the house. I don't let this stop me, I just chop and change bits, or leave them out altogether. You're not trying to win MasterChef, you just want something healthy and edible-verging-on-tasty most evenings! I often present it '...and this is my bastardisation of goulash (or the like)'.
- Frozen food. I don't mean fishfingers (although God knows how many times these hallowed frozen digits have actually saved me), I mean frozen healthy food. As well as cutting down on food waste, ready-prepped frozen fruit, vegetables and herbs are such a time-saving, smug-making bit of sorcery. If you buy or prep chopped frozen onion, garlic and ginger, you have the immediate base ingredients for a stir-fry or curry. Cubed celery, carrot and onion are the base for soup. Frozen spinach can be added to pretty much anything and makes you feel 100% healthier in a nanosecond. Frozen berries can be added to smoothies. I could go on. I am 100% a convert to frozen fruit and veg (can you tell?) as it retains all of the same nutritional value and it won't go bad and end up in the bin. If only they'd get rid of the pesky plastic wrapping, I could really polish my halo.
- I know quite a few mothers who use those 'pre-prepped' fresh food delivery services (Hello Fresh and Gousto are two that I know of). I have not tried them yet, but they are great for getting healthy food quickly, introducing variety, and cutting down on food waste.
- Look at the ingredients on packages of food. Generally, the longer the ingredients list, the further removed it is from being fresh and natural and the more likely it is to contain stuff that's not great for our system. I *do* eat stuff from packets, but I keep a weather-eye on suspect ingredients that I can't pronounce, and don't know what they are. For example I like my crisps to contain three ingredients: potato, oil, salt.

Remember that eating well is not just about maintaining a healthy weight, it is also about nourishing yourself and *enjoying* food – if that's your thing. I guess, for some, food is simply fuel – not me though! I think about food from the minute I wake up and I plan my lunch while I am eating my breakfast. I *love* food. My idea of heaven is a big gathering with everyone sharing bowls and small plates of food. However, in the long shadow of the Covid-19 pandemic, I fully understand if people prefer me to keep my thieving, germy little hands to myself. LOLz. So, yes, I love food but I want what I put in my body to be good stuff, as much as possible, and I want it to support my health rather than working against me.

## CHANGE YOUR POOPING HABITS

No one really likes to talk about poo or pooping. But here I am, taking one for the team. To read about how to have the perfect poop, go back to page 80. Essentially, hydrate, eat enough fibre, and get yourself into a more effective 'squat' position on the throne by using a step of some sort. Constipation is not only a pain in the butt, it can adversely affect your pelvic health long term. A woman who is dedicating her life to people pooping better (it's a dirty job, but someone's gotta do it!) is Dr Marisol Teijeiro, a naturopath AKA 'The Queen of Thrones'. She swears by castor oil packs, applied to the tummy area, to help get things moving. She sells these packs online, but you can also make them up yourself.

*Making a castor oil pack*
- Fold a large flannel (undyed wool or cotton) until you have a few layers.
- In a dish pour tablespoons of castor oil over the flannel until it is saturated – this is your 'pack'.
- Lay down on a large towel to avoid mess.
- Place the castor oil pack on the stomach area. Placing it on the right is said to aid the liver's function too.
- Place a small plastic sheet or some sort of old scarf that you can secure around you over the castor oil pack. This helps to heat it and press it against your skin.
- Place a hot water bottle or pad on top of the plastic/scarf to add

further heat. Make sure you don't end up with the hot water bottle touching your skin though, as this could scald.

- Leave the pack on for about an hour.

Apparently, castor oil can penetrate the skin and encourage the small intestine to push down your poop. There appears to be a lot of anecdotal evidence on this, and castor oil's therapeutic properties have been used for thousands of years, but clinical trial data is scarce – although I did find a trial in the elderly suffering with constipation which did report a significant improvement.[87]

Don't use these packs if you are pregnant.

## DO YOUR RESEARCH AND EXPLORE YOUR OPTIONS

We've given you quite a lot of information and pointers in this book, but it is not exhaustive (it was never meant to be: what mother – let alone a postpartum woman – has the time to wade through a massive tome?). There is so much more information you can access – whether online or via your GP and healthcare team – and so many experts willingly sharing their knowledge. If you are weeing too frequently, you may want to approach a urogynaecologist or women's health physio about bladder training; if you have tried pelvic floor exercises and therapy and are still having prolapse symptoms that interfere with your life, you may want to chat with a surgeon about your options; if you are suffering with vaginal dryness, hair loss that doesn't let up or intense fatigue you may want to get your hormones checked. There are almost always options for addressing any physical challenge, so it is worth finding out about what paths you can take, and how other women have managed it. I'm sorry if you're not on social media (but I definitely understand, as it can be such a time and energy drain!), as I mention quite a lot of resources that are available online, but there really is a wealth of information out there – from experts sharing their wisdom to women with lived experience, sharing their healing stories and also campaigning for change. If you have an issue, and you type the hashtag (this # symbol, followed by a word or phrase. For example: #diastasisrecti) into Twitter or Instagram, you will find so many posts come up. Be careful where you source you information though. Where possible, ensure there is a robust evidence base (from reputable and recognisable sources) and that you do not succumb to marketing for fads or get drawn into anyone peddling conspiracy theories, or, indeed, anyone who leaves you coming away feeling more negative than positive. Of course, as I've said before, forums where women share their lived experience also often fill gaps where there is no *clinical* evidence base.

If social media and the internet isn't for you, you can ask your GP for referrals or even signposting to local support groups – or maybe set up your own, as Helen Lauer did when she was struggling with being diagnosed with a prolapse. Helen found that 'the power of women who understand what you're going through is incredible. Even with a small group, each of us had such different experiences, yet gained so much from the group. It encouraged a few group members to address problems they had been "just dealing with", instead of getting proper care and input'. Your library should also be able to order you in any book that you think would help expand your understanding of your body, your hormones and your overall health. World of Books is also a great resource for buying second-hand books. With any of this, if the first door you knock on doesn't open, or the person behind it does not properly address your needs, walk up the road and try the next one, and the next… until you are content. As well as building villages to support us in the job of mothering, we need to build support networks for our health. Find your tribe – and don't give up if it takes some time.

## DON'T FORGET JOY

While writing this book, I have been through many ups and downs. In my own life, but also through the experiences of women who (sometimes avoidably) suffered throughout their postpartum transitions. But at no point have I regretted pregnancy, at no point have I regretted birth, at no point have I regretted being a mother. Why? Because, along with the rough bits, there is immense joy to be had in motherhood. Not only that, but remember, when looking at statistics, there are large numbers of women who are *not* adversely affected. If 50% of women end up with some form of prolapse (and remember, this may even be asymptomatic for many), then 50% do *not* end up with prolapse. That's a lot of women. With continence statistics, even if they were at the worse end of estimates, that's still hundreds of thousands of women every year who do *not* have continence issues. If one in 10 women suffer with postnatal depression, then nine in 10 do not. And so on. As awareness grows about prenatal and perinatal empowerment and health, and the support needed to enable women and birthing people to thrive is put in place, these figures will also hopefully come down. I read a really powerful message from a husband to a wife, as she was lamenting the changes to her body after childbirth. He texted her, 'what if you just loved her today?'. The 'her' being her body. A body that she felt was battered and broken. So, she did. She shelved punishing exercise routines and paused the negative feedback loop in her brain and just loved and nourished her body. Your body does stuff throughout pregnancy that is mind-blowing. It heals as best it can and then it meets the challenges of parenting day in and day out, regardless of which bits work and which don't. If that isn't deserving of a bit of love today, then I don't know what is.

*Side note:* regret and motherhood are words you will not often see together. That said, regret should not come with the side dish of shame that it currently does. If you *do* have regrets, this does not make you either a bad human or a bad mother. It is possible to love your children *and* regret becoming a mother. It's fucking hard work and can test your mind and body to their limits. You are far from alone in this.

## AND A NOTE ON BIRTH

Birth can be beautiful. Even though neither of my births was a walk in the park, I have fond memories from both experiences. From powering through the 'surges' (yes, I'm one of 'them') in my first birth to listening to Bob Marley while I lay, clutching my husband's hand, on the operating table with my second, there are moments I will never forget, and that I cherish. The moments when I was handed my sons are two of the most transcendental and life-affirming I have ever experienced. While an uncomplicated birth cannot be guaranteed for everyone, there are moves towards creating better environments to facilitate this, and beautiful birth experiences are not fairy stories. If you seek out positive birth stories, you will find them. Fear and anxiety are not conducive to calm, uncomplicated births, so, where possible – and when you've got all your plans in place to aid your recovery – tune out of everything else so that your brain and body may relax.

## AND HOPE

There is a lot going on for us, both as we age, and as our body recovers and adapts to motherhood, and it can be overwhelming. But if researching this book has taught me one thing, it is that there is a huge push happening in women's health at the moment and a wealth of extremely well-equipped health practitioners trying to spread awareness and effect change. There was a review of maternity services in 2016 and, as a result, a National Maternity Transformation Partnership was established which is working hard on rectifying some of the issues raised in this book. It won't be quick work, and so, in the meantime, I do implore you to do your research, listen to your body and seek help (and keep going when you hit brick walls), and reach out to find others who have been through something similar so that you can support each other. Despite some of the more difficult stories and experiences relayed in this book, I feel very hopeful for the future of women's health and the mothers that come after us.

## AND FINALLY...

Whenever I read a non-fiction book, there is always one thing which stays with me. My hope is that the one thing you take from this book is this: *you matter*.

# TOP TIPS FROM
# THE EXPERTS

Dr Rebecca Moore, consultant perinatal psychiatrist, is wary of giving 'top tips' as everyone is so unique, and their personal circumstances so individual, that it would not speak to everyone reading. She never prescribes the same treatment plan twice in her practice and she also feels that women can be overwhelmed with shame or guilt if they cannot act on advice given to them. I am including this in this section as it is worth bearing in mind: what works for someone else may not work for you – and that's OK.

*'Be pro-active and co-design your recovery with your healthcare providers.'* Professor Debra Bick OBE, professor of clinical trials in maternal health

*'Don't "just put up with it". If a bit of you hurts, or leaks, or isn't quite right then take it to see a GP or a pelvic health physio. It takes an average of seven years for a woman to seek help for stress incontinence, which is a shame because most cases improve, or are cured, with treatment.'* Elaine Miller, pelvic physiotherapist and comedian

*'Pain should not be part of the postnatal package. Why maternity normalises it beggars belief. If pain is limiting normal activities, it needs to be addressed. Recognise when to seek help, as it can impact both mother and baby.'* Dr Sunita Sharma, obstetrician-gynaecologist

*'Do pelvic floor exercises as often as possible both during pregnancy and after birth. These can provide not only short-term benefits postnatally, but long-term benefits around the menopause and beyond.'* Dr Eloise Elphinstone, GP

*'Now starts a new chapter of your life, proceed with empathy for you and your body. Take your time, have patience as your body heals and remember to just breathe.'* Sundas Khalid, midwife

'*Move in a way that brings you joy.*' Kim Vopni, restorative exercise specialist

'*Don't feel guilty if you feel you are eating in unhealthy ways, just think about why you're eating the way you are and add to your plate next time. Don't focus on what to remove, instead add more colour, more fibre, more nutrients. Also, don't look at one day, or even one week, as a picture of how you're doing. It is not the whole picture. Take a longer view and be gentle with yourself. Maybe next week you'll eat a tonne of fruit and vegetables. Understand why you do things so you can make small changes without beating yourself up about it.*' Jo Sharp, nutritionist

'*Take it slow with sex and focus on intimacy. Most of all, have fun.*' Sam Evans, sexual health expert

'*Eat lots of protein and carbohydrate-rich vegetables, for the B-vitamins. Hair is made of protein. If you're not eating it, you can't make new hair.*' Sally-Ann Tarver, trichologist

'*Don't be ashamed. If [bowel] symptoms persist – seek help.*' Julie Cornish, colorectal surgeon

'*Don't forget about yourself. Nourish your body using simple plate building guidance: ½ plate of veggies; ¼ plate of protein and ¼ plate of complex carbs. Keep things simple and enjoy wholesome foods.*' Eva Johnson, nutritionist

'*The resting time postpartum is deeply restorative for your body to recover, your mind to adjust to the birth and new role, and your soul to connect with the new life you have brought into the world.*' Tracey Allport, occupational and complementary therapist

'*Only you know what's normal for you: we can feel so uncertain in the early days of parenting and question whether what we're feeling is ok. Often we minimise our concerns and they can be overlooked or dismissed as 'new parent worries'. While this is a whole new world, you know yourself best so do seek support if you're not feeling how you want to be feeling.*' Dr Emma Svanberg, clinical psychologist

*'Get as much rest as you can in the weeks following birth. This means asking for plenty of help from friends and family or hiring help if that's affordable. This period of rest will leave the mum feeling less depleted in the long run as they will have had the chance to heal from birth and honour this huge transition into parenthood.'* Laura Rice, doula

*'Pregnancy is a stress test for life, if you have issues/ complications during pregnancy then these type of issues may potentially resurface later in life. Be proactive.'* Dr Iona Thorne, rheumatologist

*'Keeping milk moving is really the best way for your breasts to stay healthy and well. Look outside of yourself for help if you're struggling to breastfeed.'* Lucy Ruddle, lactation consultant

*'I would advise postpartum women to follow their maternal instincts, trust that their brains have been fine-tuned to care for their babies, give in to their maternal drive and try to enjoy this unique period as much as possible.'* Dr Elseline Hoekzema, neuroscientist

*'Give yourself time to heal, give yourself the support and care you need to recover and if something doesn't feel right to you within your body… please seek help!'* Edel McCann, women's health physiotherapist

*'Understand the changes your body has gone through and be realistic with your expectations of yourself. And don't let anyone tell you that your experience doesn't matter, it's important to be heard.'* Gemma Dawson, osteopath, Mummy MOT practitioner and Pilates instructor

*'You might have lots of preconceived ideas about what parenthood looks like and it can be a shock to find out that it's actually very different to your expectations. Be kind to yourself. Keep it simple and prioritise connection. And know that every single on of us is winging it. You've got this.'* Anna Le Grange, mindful breastfeeding counsellor

'It's so hard to do but ask for help so that you can get some rest; or ask for help with your mental health if you're struggling after a difficult birth experience or struggling with the transition to life as a parent. Remember your baby doesn't need a perfect parent, they just need you! So drop your own expectations of yourself and give yourself a break!' Sophie Hiscock, midwife

'Be as honest and open as you can with yourself and others about your feelings and needs. Know that whatever you're feeling is okay. When we're struggling, we often feel alone and blame ourselves, but it's not just you and it's not your fault. Your feelings are a natural response to your circumstances, and they're there to give you some clues about what you might need.' Catherine Topham Sly, counsellor

'Prioritise your recovery in the early days – rest in the first few weeks and then make sure you are mobilising your body, especially your pelvis. Try to go for walks regularly, book in for specialist Pilates classes (or find an expert online and do their videos), go and see a women's health physio or women's health osteopath and see these things as non-negotiable.' Grace Lillywhite, Pilates teacher

'Never underestimate what good oral home care can do for your oral and general health. The mouth is the gateway to the whole body, taking care of it with good brushing, flossing and dental visits will mean your body is able to recover postnatally, to provide for your newborn and maintain your own long-term health.' Lottie Manahan, dental hygienist

Lyanne Nicholl (me): Don't write a book!

# FURTHER READING
# AND RESOURCES

## BOOKS

Brathwaite, C. *I am not your Baby Mother*, Quercus, 2020

Brown, A. *Let's talk about... feeding your baby*, Pinter & Martin, 2021

Enders, G. *Gut*, Scribe UK, 2017

Hayes, A. *The Supermum Myth: Become a happier mum by overcoming anxiety, ditching guilt and embracing imperfection using CBT and mindfulness techniques*, White Ladder Press, 2017

Hill, M. *The Positive Birth Book: A New Approach to Pregnancy, Birth and the Early Weeks (revised and updated second edition)*, Pinter & Martin, 2022

Hill, M. *Period Power – Harness Your Hormones and Get Your Cycle Working For You*, Green Tree, 2019

Hill, M. *Perimenopause Power: Navigating your hormones on the journey to menopause*, Green Tree, 2021

Hogenboom, M. *The Motherhood Complex: The Story of Our Changing Selves*, Piatkus, 2021

Messager, S. *Why Postnatal Recovery Matters*, Pinter & Martin, 2020

McNish, H. *Nobody Told Me – Poetry and Parenthood*, Fleet, 2020

Nagoski, E. *Come as you are: the bestselling guide to the new science that will transform your sex life: 1*, Scribe UK, 2015

Ou, H. *The First Forty Days*, Stewart, Tabori & Chang, 2016

Perel, E. *Mating in Captivity: Unlocking erotic intelligence*, Yellow Kite, 2017

Ryan, M. *Baby Bod*, Baby Bod Press, 2015

Sellerach, O. *The Postnatal Depletion Cure*, Sphere, 2018

Simpson, J. *The Pelvic Floor Bible: Everything You Need to Know to Prevent and Cure Problems at Every Stage in Your Life*, Penguin Life, 2019

Schiller, R *Your No Guilt Pregnancy Plan: A revolutionary guide to pregnancy, birth and the weeks that follow*, Penguin Life, 2018

Strickland, A. and Hands, B. *The Little Book of Self-Care for New Mums*, Vermilion, 2018

Svanberg, E. *Why Birth Trauma Matters* Pinter & Martin, 2019
Uvnäs-Moberg, K. *Why Oxytocin Matters*, Pinter & Martin, 2019
Yate, Z. *When Breastfeeding Sucks: What you need to know about nursing aversion and agitation*, Pinter & Martin, 2020

## PHYSICAL HEALTH RESOURCES

Centred Mums (Pilates) – www.centredmums.com
Bettina Rae (Yoga) – www.bettinarae.com
Honest Yoga – www.honestyoga.co.uk
Mutu System – www.mutusystem.com
Holistic Core Restore – www.holisticcorerestore.com
Pelvic Floor Recovery – www.pelvicfloorrecovery.com
Institute for Birth Healing – www.instituteforbirthhealing.com
Vagina Coach – www.vaginacoach.com
The Physio Mummy – www.physiomummy.com
MASIC Foundation - www.masic.org.uk
Caesarean recovery – www.hannahjohnsontherapies.com
Diastasis recovery – mybumpbirthandbeyond.tumblr.com
Dr Janelle Howell – www.vaginarehabdoctor.com
Private pelvic health physios – www.themummymot.com

## MENTAL HEALTH RESOURCES

PANDAS Foundation for Pre And Postnatal Depression Advice and Support: www.pandasfoundation.org.uk and 0808 1961 776 (10am–11pm every day)
Action on Postpartum Psychosis: www.app-network.org
MIND www.mind.org.uk
Birth Trauma Association www.birthtraumaassociation.org.uk
Make Birth Better www.makebirthbetter.org.uk
Home Start – www.home-start.org.uk
Perinatal Mental Health Partnership:
    Instagram @perinatalmhpartnership
The Motherhood Group: www.themotherhoodgroup.com
Birth Debrief Facilitator – Instagram @mixing.up.motherhood
Help for Traveller, Gypsy and Roma communities
    www.travellermovement.org.uk

## PREGNANCY AND BABY LOSS, STILLBIRTH AND NEONATAL DEATH RESOURCES

The Miscarriage Association – www.miscarriageassociation.org.uk
Nova Foundation – www.novafoundation.org.uk
Tommys – www.tommys.org
Sands – www.sands.org.uk
Aching Arms – www.achingarms.co.uk
Leos – www.leosneonatal.org

## PREMATURE BABIES AND UNWELL BABIES

Bliss – www.bliss.org.uk
The NICU Mummy – www.nicumummy.co.uk

## LGBTQI

Queer Birth Club www.queerbirthclub.org.uk
Pink Parents www.pinkparents.org.uk

## PREGNANCY, BIRTH AND POSTPARTUM SUPPORT

NCT – www.nct.org.uk
Daisy Foundation – www.thedaisyfoundation.com
Doula UK – www.doula.org.uk
Doulas Without Borders – www.doulaswithoutborders.com
Abuela Doulas – www.abueladoulas.co.uk
Birthrights – www.birthrights.org.uk
Best Beginnings – www.bestbeginnings.org.uk
Association of South Asian Midwives – www.asamidwives.co.uk
Beyond Birth Living Library – www.beyondbirthlivinglibrary.org
Menopause – www.newsonhealth.co.uk
Nutrition – www.sharpnutrition.co.uk and www.eva-johnson.com
Sex toys and lubricants – www.jodivine.com
Breastfeeding – www.laleche.org.uk and www.lucyruddle.co.uk and www.mindfulbreastfeeding.co.uk
Autoimmune and rare disease organisations – www.aimscharity.org and www.raredisease.org.uk
Single mothers – www.gingerbread.org.uk
Disabled parents – Instagram @_beyondstrength_
Mum and Tea - mumsandtea.com

# ACKNOWLEDGEMENTS

Firstly, thank you to Rebecca Schiller for the initial encouragement and guidance. Huge thanks to all of the women, over the years, who have shared their birth, postnatal and pregnancy/baby loss experiences with me. I hope this book adequately reflects your feelings and hopes for change. To the women (and man!) who gave their time to come to Parliament in 2018, hosted by Rosie Duffield, to push for improvements in postnatal care. To the other campaigning groups and individuals that continue to push for change in this area.

This book would not have been written without the frank testimonial and the expertise of all the women quoted within. I am humbled that you trusted me with your stories and words of wisdom. To The Loomies (mad but wonderful bunch that you are), the Grazia Readers (in particular Dr Meera Sood), the Tooting Massive and the Lockdown Littlies groups for your honesty, insight and wit. In particular, thanks to advance readers Sabrina Sweeney and Dr Emily Lau. Thank you to Abby Hollick for allowing me to borrow bits from the Postnatal FAQ podcast. Thank you to all my friends far and wide who have been so encouraging – even the ones who are slightly bewildered by 'all this'. Thank you, especially, to mega legend Kristy MacLeod and also to Claire Barlow for your constant support and your inspiring attitude to recovery. Thank you to advance readers Anna Whitehouse, Emma Haslett, Sabrina Sweeney and Dr Emily Lau.

Thank you to the women of Whitstable for supporting and sustaining me, in many different ways, including Jo Jell at The Workspace on the Farm, Mel Keat at The Worker's League (I'll never forget that gin and relief!), Gemma Dawson (for starting this journey with me), Nina Bainbridge, Helen Sansom, Katy Oliver, Lucy Browne, Pam Pittman, Rhiannon Newson, Emma Mayo and all my fellow sea-dippers and oat latte sippers.

Thank you to our NHS healthcare workers. Although there are examples of poor care reported in this book, it remains a fact that our beloved institution is run mostly on the goodwill and commitment of many extraordinary individuals who go above and beyond the call of duty to try and provide great care while working under intolerable conditions. Vote wisely, dear readers.

Thank you Pinter & Martin (particularly my editor, Susan Last) for taking a chance on me and dealing with all of my rookie writer angst. Creating this with the backdrop of a pandemic and playing whack-a-mole with sick kids has been quite the endurance test.

Thank you to my family for being excellent cheerleaders. Especially Mum for always being open about pregnancy loss and Donna for showing me that you can try, try, try again. Thank you Dad (now departed) for showing me the joy of putting pen to paper, and the commitment needed to keep going. Thanks to my beastie boys for the light relief, and for showing me pure love and joy – I'd do it all again for you. And finally, Richard Nicholl – for always being in my corner.

# ABOUT THE AUTHOR

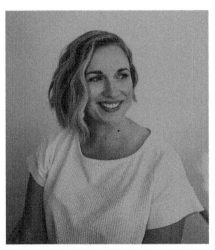

author photo Abigail Watson

Lyanne Nicholl trained and worked as an actor before establishing a career in the charity sector. Lyanne has spent the last 15 years working with small and medium-sized charities, helping them with fundraising, research and copywriting. After the birth of her first child, Lyanne became interested in postnatal care – or the lack thereof – and began campaigning work which led to the idea for her first book *Your Postnatal Body*. After experiencing recurrent miscarriage, Lyanne was thrilled to welcome her second child. Not so thrilling was that he arrived two weeks before the Covid pandemic struck the UK and 'confinement' took on a whole new meaning. Lyanne lives on the East Kent coast with her husband and two sons, writing and doing consultancy work for charities.

# PANJEERI RECIPE

*(see page 44)*

Sundas Khalid: *The following recipe is my grandmother's recipe but you can substitute some of the nuts she used for your own choice, e.g. hazelnuts, pistachios, brazil nuts etc. You can even increase the amounts of coconut/raisins or anything really as per your own taste.*

### Ingredients

- ½ cup almonds
- ½ cup cashews
- ½ cup walnuts
- ½ cup lotus seeds (phool makhana)
- ½ cup melon seeds (charmagaz)
- ½ cup flakes or desiccated coconut
- ½ cup oats ( can use coarse wheat)
- ½ cup sesame seeds
- ¼ cup sunflower seeds
- ¼ cup pumpkin seeds
- ¼ cup gond (gum arabic)
- 2tbsp whole flaxseeds
- ½ - ¼ cup raisins (can be adjusted to personal preference)
- 1 cup semolina (sooji)
- Ghee, as needed
- ½ cup sweetener of choice (white sugar, brown sugar, coconut sugar, gurr, shakkar etc), powdered (grind it in a grinder)

### Instructions

1. Heat 2 tbsp of ghee in a pot or pan. Top the ghee up as needed, whenever it is about to finish.
2. Start by frying the almonds over a medium/low heat. Fry these until they are fragrant. Remove with a slotted spoon and set aside in a large bowl.
3. Add the cashews into the ghee. Fry until light brown and fragrant. Set aside in the large bowl alongside the almonds.
4. Add the walnuts into the ghee. Fry until slightly change colour and

fragrant. Set aside with the other nuts.

5. Add the lotus seeds (phool makhana) to the ghee. These absorb a lot of ghee. Fry until they change colour and crunchy and not like popcorn, it's done. Set aside with the other nuts.

6. Add the melon seeds to the ghee. Fry until golden and fragrant. Set aside with the other nuts.

7. Add the coconut to the ghee. This will begin to brown VERY quickly. Remove and set aside with the other nuts.

8. Add the oats to the ghee. Fry until golden brown – this takes about ten minutes. Remove and set aside with the other nuts.

9. Add the sesame seeds to the ghee. Fry until golden brown and fragrant. Remove and set aside with the other nuts.

10. Add the sunflower seeds to the ghee. Fry until brown and fragrant. Remove and set aside with the other nuts.

11. Add the pumpkin seeds to the ghee. Fry until brown and fragrant. Remove and set aside with the other nuts.

12. Add the gond (gum arabic) to the ghee. Fry these until they become puffy and stop spluttering. IF THESE TURN VERY HARD, DO NOT ADD THESE TO THE NUT MIXTURE.

13. Add the flaxseeds to the ghee. Fry for 3-4 minutes, Remove and set aside with the other nuts.

14. Add the raisins to the ghee. Fry till they swell – this happens VERY quickly so be careful. Remove and set these in a SEPARATE bowl from the other nuts.

15. Add the semolina (sooji) to the ghee. Fry this well, stirring often until it becomes brown and fragrant. This can take upto 10 minutes on low heat. Remove and set this aside with the raisins.

16. Now put all the nuts and seeds in a food processor and grind the mixture coarsely.

17. Stir in the fried raisins, semolina and powdered sugar, gurr or sweetener of your choice you can adjust the sugar to taste.

Store in an air-tight container in a cool place. This has a rather long shelf life, but ideally consume within 4-6 weeks.

© Nabila Khalid

# REFERENCES

1 'Oxytocin in Pregnancy and the Postpartum: Relations to Labor and Its Management' Marie Prevost, Phyllis Zelkowitz, Togas Tulandi, Barbara Hayton, Nancy Feeley, C. Sue Carter, Lawrence Joseph, Hossein Pournajafi-Nazarloo, Erin Yong Ping, Haim Abenhaim, and Ian Gold, 2014

2 'Prospective evaluation of night time hot flashes during pregnancy and postpartum' Rebecca C Thurston, James F Luther, Stephen R Wisniewski, Heather Eng, Katherine L Wisner, 2013

3 'Postpartum Headache' Kathleen J Richardson, 2017

4 https://www.nhs.uk/conditions/pre-eclampsia/treatment/

5 https://www.rcoa.ac.uk/sites/default/files/documents/2019-11/10-HeadachesSpinalEpiduralweb.pdf

6 https://www.nhs.uk/conditions/irritable-bowel-syndrome-ibs/further-help-and-support/

7 'Dysphoric milk ejection reflex: A case report' Alia M Heise and Diane Wiessinger, 2011

8 'Dysphoric Milk Ejection Reflex: A Descriptive Study' Tamara L Ureño, Cristóbal S Berry-Cabán, Ashley Adams, Toni L Buchheit, Susan G Hopkinson, 2019

9 'Pregnancy leads to long-lasting changes in human brain structure' Elseline Hoekzema, Erika Barba-Müller, Cristina Pozzobon, Marisol Picado, Florencio Lucco, David García-García, Juan Carlos Soliva, Adolf Tobeña, Manuel Desco, Eveline A Crone, Agustín Ballesteros, Susanna Carmona and Oscar Vilarroya, 2016

10 Brain plasticity in pregnancy and the postpartum period: links to maternal caregiving and mental health, Erika Barba-Müller, Sinéad Craddock, Susanna Carmona & Elseline Hoekzema, 2018

11 'The maternal brain and its plasticity in humans' Pilyoung Kim, Lane Strathearn, James E Swain, 2016

12 'Metabolic, Endocrine, and Immune Consequences of Sleep Deprivation' Laila AlDabal and Ahmed S BaHammam, 2011

13 'Changes in gustatory function during the course of pregnancy and postpartum' Nicole Ochsenbein-Kölble, Ruth von Mering, Roland Zimmermann, Thomas Hummel, 2005

14 'Voice pitch modulation in human mate choice' Katarzyna Pisanski, Anna Oleszkiewicz, Justyna Plachetka, Marzena Gmiterek and David Reby, 2018

15 'Oral and dental health care practices in pregnant women in Australia: a postnatal survey' Natalie J Thomas, Philippa F Middleton and

Caroline A Crowther, 2008

16 'Does the rate of orthodontic tooth movement change during pregnancy and lactation? A systematic review of the evidence from animal studies' Moaza Omar, Eleftherios G Kaklamanos, 2020

17 'Vitamin B12 deficiency among patients with diabetes mellitus: is routine screening and supplementation justified?' Davis Kibirige, Raymond Mwebaze, 2013

18 https://www.nhs.uk/conditions/vitamin-b12-or-folate-deficiency-anaemia/causes/

19 'Melasma' Hajira Basit , Kiran V. Godse, Ahmad M. Al Aboud 2020

20 'The clinical importance of visceral adiposity: a critical review of methods for visceral adipose tissue analysis' A Shuster, M Patlas, J H Pinthus, M Mourtzakis, 2012

21 'Prevalence and risk factors of diastasis recti abdominis from late pregnancy to 6 months postpartum, and relationship with lumbo-pelvic pain' Patrícia Gonçalves Fernandes da Mota, Augusto Gil Brites Andrade Pascoal, Ana Isabel Andrade Dinis Carita, Kari Bø, 2014

22 'Phantom Kicks': Women's Subjective Experience of Foetal Kicks after the Postpartum Period' Disha Sasan, Phillip GD Ward, Meredith Nash, Edwina R Orchard, Michael J Farrell, Jakob Hohwy, Sharna Jamadar, 2019

23 'Prospective study of intraabdominal adhesions among women of different races with or without keloids' Togas Tulandi, Baydaa Al-Sannan, Ghadeer Akbar, Cleve Ziegler, Louise Miner, 2011

24 'Incisional endometriosis: A rare cause for a painful scar – A report and commentary' Brijesh K Biswas, Nalini Gupta, Navneet Magon, 2012

25 https://patient.info/doctor/postpartum-endometritis-pro

26 'Piriformis syndrome occurring after pregnancy' Ali Kemal Sivrioglu, Selahattin Ozyurek, Hakan Mutlu, and Guner Sonmez, 2013

27 'Predictors and consequences of long-term pregnancy-related pelvic girdle pain: a longitudinal follow-up study' Helen Elden, Annelie Gutke, Gunilla Kjellby-Wendt, Monika Fagevik-Olsen and Hans-Christian Ostgaard, 2016

28 'Can incontinence be cured? A systematic review of cure rates' Rob Riemsma, Suzanne Hagen, Ruth Kirschner-Hermanns, Christine Norton, Helle Wijk, Karl-Erik Andersson, Christopher Chapple, Julian Spinks, Adrian Wagg, Edward Hutt, Kate Misso, Sohan Deshpande, Jos Kleijnen and Ian Milsom, 2017

29 'Postpartum period three distinct but continuous phases' Mattea Romano, Alessandra Cacciatore, Rosalba Giordano, and Beatrice La Rosa, 2010

30 'Prevalence, incidence and bothersomeness of urinary incontinence between 6 weeks and 1 year post-partum: a systematic review

and meta-analysis' Heidi F.A. Moossdorff-Steinhauser, Bary C.M. Berghmans, Marc E.A. Spaanderman, and Esther M.J. Bols, 2021

31  'Prevalence and risk factors for pelvic organ prolapse 20 years after childbirth: a national cohort study in singleton primiparae after vaginal or caesarean delivery' M Gyhagen, M Bullarbo, T.F.Nielsen, I. Milsom, 2012

32  'Vaginal childbirth and pelvic floor disorders' Hafsa U Memon, Victoria L Handa, 2013/Yenial et al, 2013

33  'Prolapse and sexual function in women with benign joint hypermobility syndrome' H Mastoroudes, I Giarenis,L Cardozo, S Srikrishna, M Vella, D Robinson, H Kazkaz, R Grahame, 2012

34  'Dyspareunia and childbirth: a prospective cohort study' E A McDonald, D Gartland, R Small, S J Brown, 2015

35  'Sonographic finding of postpartum levator ani muscle injury correlates with pelvic floor clinical examination' M Lipschuetz, D V Valsky, L Shick-Naveh, H Daum, B Messing, I Yagel, S Yagel, S M Cohen, 2014

36  'Obstetric factors associated with levator ani muscle injury after vaginal birth' Rohna Kearney, Janis M Miller, James A Ashton-Miller, John O L DeLancey, 2006

37  'Clinical consequences of levator trauma' H.P. Dietz, 2012

38  Kubotani et al, 2020

39  https://www.nhs.uk/common-health-questions/pregnancy/when-will-my-periods-start-again-after-pregnancy/

40  'Pregnancy leads to lasting changes in foot structure' Neil A Segal, Elizabeth R Boyer, Patricia Teran-Yengle, Natalie A Glass, Howard J Hillstrom, H John Yack, 2013

41  'Fetal microchimerism and maternal health: A review and evolutionary analysis of cooperation and conflict beyond the womb' Amy M. Boddy, Angelo Fortunato, Melissa Wilson Sayres, Athena Aktipis, 2015

42  'Can women correctly contract their pelvic floor muscles without formal instruction?' J. Welles Henderson, MD, Siqing Wang, MD, MS, MStat, Marlene J Egger, PhD, Professor, Maria Masters, RN, and Ingrid Nygaard, MD, MS, Professor, 2013

43  'The role of massage in scar management: a literature review' Thuzar M Shin 1, Jeremy S Bordeaux, 2011

44  'Physical Management of Scar Tissue: A Systematic Review and Meta-Analysis' Carlina Deflorin, Erich Hohenauer, Rahel Stoop, Ulrike van Daele, Ron Clijsen, and Jan Taeymans, 2020

45  'Comparison of pelvic floor dysfunction 6 years after uncomplicated vaginal versus elective cesarean deliveries: a cross-sectional study' David Baud, Joanna Sichitiu, Valeria Lombardi, Maud De Rham, Sylvain Meyer, Yvan Vial and Chahin Achtari, 2020

46 https://abuhb.nhs.wales/files/physiotherapy/perineal-scar-massage-pdf/
47 Schummers et al, 2018
48 'Comparison of the effect of ginger and zinc sulfate on primary dysmenorrhea: a placebo-controlled randomized trial' Farzaneh Kashefi, Marjan Khajehei, Mahbubeh Tabatabaeichehr, Mohammad Alavinia, Javad Asili, 2014
49 https://www.absolute.physio/wp-content/uploads/2019/09/returning-to-running-postnatal-guidelines.pdf
50 https://www.nhs.uk/live-well/exercise/couch-to-5k-week-by-week/
51 'Genital Prolapse Surgery: What Options Do We Have in the Age of Mesh Issues?' Guenter K. Noé, 2021
52 'Caesarean section and risk for endometriosis: a prospective cohort study of Swedish registries' Andolf E, Thorsell M, Källén K. 2013
53 'Skin Endometriosis at the Caesarean Section Scar: A Case Report and Review of the Literature' Monitoring Editor: Alexander Muacevic and John R Adler, 2018
54 https://www.diabetes.org.uk/diabetes-the-basics/gestational-diabetes
55 Mayo Clinic
56 https://www.bhf.org.uk/what-we-do/news-from-the-bhf/news-archive/2019/june/high-blood-pressure-during-pregnancy-increases-risk-of-heart-attacks-and-strokes | https://www.cdc.gov/bloodpressure/pregnancy
57 As above
58 'Sex differences in autoimmune disease from a pathological perspective' DeLisa Fairweather 1, Sylvia Frisancho-Kiss, Noel R Rose, 2008
59 'Postpartum autoimmune thyroid syndrome: a model of aggravation of autoimmune disease' N Amino 1, H Tada, Y Hidaka, 1999
60  www.fivexmore.com
61 'A clinical update on hypermobile Ehlers-Danlos syndrome during pregnancy, birth and beyond' Sally Pezaro, Gemma Pearce and Emma Reinhold, 2021
62 Mother and Babies: Reducing Risk Through Audits and Confidential Enquiries across the UK
63 https://www.kingsfund.org.uk/publications/health-people-ethnic-minority-groups-england
64 https://www.vice.com/en/article/jgxne7/nima-bhakta-suicide-from-postpartum-depression-is-a-reminder-to-remove-mental-health-stigma-in-south-asia
65 'The delay of motherhood: Reasons, determinants, time used to achieve pregnancy, and maternal anxiety level' Leticia Molina-García, Manuel Hidalgo-Ruiz, Eva María Cocera-Ruíz, Esther Conde-Puertas, Miguel

Delgado-Rodríguez, Juan Miguel Martínez-Galiano, 2019

66 'Association of Parity and Breastfeeding With Risk of Early Natural Menopause' Christine R. Langton, Brian W. Whitcomb, Alexandra C. Purdue-Smithe, Lynnette L. Sievert, Susan E. Hankinson, JoAnn E. Manson, Bernard A. Rosner, and Elizabeth R. Bertone-Johnson, 2020

67 www.millionwomenstudy.org

68 https://www.cancerresearchuk.org/about-cancer/causes-of-cancer/hormones-and-cancer/does-hormone-replacement-therapy-increase-cancer-risk

69 'Postmenopausal women are at risk of urogynaecological dysfunction. With better understanding of the pelvic floor, much can be done to improve care', Judith Lee, The Nursing Times, 2009

70 'Effect of oestrogen therapy on faecal incontinence in postmenopausal women' Bach, Fiona L; Sairally, B Zeyah F; Latthe, Pallavi, 2018

71 https://www.bbc.co.uk/programmes/articles/1mW6885X3N2gKnVjXT00KCj/how-to-reset-your-brain-with-your-breathing

72 'Improve postoperative sleep: what can we do?' Xian Su 1, Dong-Xin Wang, 2018

73 'Provision About Lactation After Stillbirth and Infant Death' Katherine Carroll, PhD, Debbie Noble-Carr, PhD, Lara Sweeney, Catherine Waldby, 2020

74 'Physical health problems after childbirth and maternal depression at six to seven months postpartum' S Brown, J Lumley, 2000

75 'Physical health after childbirth and maternal depression in the first 12 months post partum: results of an Australian nulliparous pregnancy cohort study' Hannah Woolhouse, Deirdre Gartland, Susan Perlen, Susan Donath, Stephanie J Brown 2014

76 'The neuroendocrinological aspects of pregnancy and postpartum depression' S. Trifu, A. Vladuti, and A. Popescu, 2019

77 https://drchatterjee.com/blog/category/stress/

78 'Can pelvic floor muscle training reverse pelvic organ prolapse and reduce prolapse symptoms? An assessor-blinded, randomized, controlled trial' Ingeborg Hoff Braekken 1, Memona Majida, Marie Ellström Engh, Kari Bø, 2010 | 'Individualised pelvic floor muscle training in women with pelvic organ prolapse (POPPY): a multicentre randomised controlled trial' Suzanne Hagen, Diane Stark, Cathryn Glazener, Sylvia Dickson, Sarah Barry, Andrew Elders, Helena Frawley, Mary P Galea, Janet Logan, Alison McDonald, Gladys McPherson, Kate H Moore, John Norrie, Andrew Walker, Don Wilson, POPPY Trial Collaborators, 2014

79 'Postdural puncture headache' Kyung-Hwa Kwak, 2017

80 https://wrisk.org/uncategorized/what-does-risk-in-pregnancy-mean-

to-you/

81 'Impact of Doulas on Healthy Birth Outcomes' Kenneth J. Gruber, Susan H. Cupito, and Christina F. Dobson, 2013

82 Above

83 'Outcomes of Care for 1,892 Doula-Supported Adolescent Births in the United States: The DONA International Data Project, 2000 to 2013' Courtney L. Everson, Melissa Cheyney, and Marit L. Bovbjerg, 2018

84 'Epidemiology and outcome assessment of pelvic organ prolapse' Matthew D Barber, Christopher Maher, 2013

85 Sharp et al, 2018

86 'Effectiveness of Acupuncture Used for the Management of Postpartum Depression: A Systematic Review and Meta-Analysis' Wei Li, Ping Yin, Lixing Lao, Shifen Xu 2018

87 'An examination of the effect of castor oil packs on constipation in the elderly' Gülşah Gürol Arslan, Ismet Eşer, 2011

# INDEX